Yoga for Pregnancy & Birth

A GUIDE FOR YOGA TEACHERS

Megan Sloan

Be Strong Yoga Publications

Seattle, WA

Copyright © 2019 by Megan Sloan.

All rights reserved. No part of this publication may be reproduced, distributed or transmitted in any form or by any means, including photocopying, recording, or other electronic or mechanical methods, without the prior written permission of the publisher, except in the case of brief quotations embodied in critical reviews and certain other noncommercial uses permitted by copyright law.

Megan Sloan/Be Strong Yoga Publications
Seattle, WA
www.bestrongmama.com

Book Layout ©2017 BookDesignTemplates.com

Yoga for Pregnancy & Birth: A Guide for Yoga Teachers/ Megan Sloan. —1st ed.
ISBN 978-1-7342195-2-4

Contents

I've learned that people will forget what you said,
people will forget what you did,
but people will never forget how you made them feel.

—MAYA ANGELOU

Introduction

I began my journey in the perinatal world in 2009 when I took my first Prenatal Yoga teacher training program. I took this training out of curiosity and a desire to work more closely with the pregnant yoga students who attended my yoga classes from time to time. I was fascinated with birth and pregnancy—though, at the time, it was hard for me to see myself ever becoming a mother. It felt far away, like something that would happen to someone else. Eyes open wide, I completely dove into this new experience of what it meant to inhabit a body that could carry and birth a child.

I started teaching Prenatal Yoga classes soon after the training and was always amazed by all the different people who would walk through my doors. Over the next 10 years, I would teach prenatal yoga to hundreds of pregnant students, watching their pregnancies unfolding, cheering them on through the experience, empathizing with the discomforts of their pregnancy, and supporting them in unexpected challenges when babies flipped breech in the last few weeks or moments of despair when a pregnancy loss occurred.

Two years into teaching prenatal yoga, I felt a strong desire to span the entirety of the perinatal experience for my students and began teaching postnatal yoga classes, as well. Postnatal classes were a whole new experience. Imagine being in a yoga class with several crying babies and an instructor trying to teach while holding one or two of them. It was chaos! But it was magical. I loved seeing new parents come in after their babies were born and reveled in meeting their little ones. It brought the whole journey full circle as I would hold these new babies in my arms after watching their parents go through nearly their entire pregnancies in my class. Each time I taught, I felt so blessed to be part of such an intimate journey—even more so when I could then hold these sweet, long-anticipated babies in my arms.

And while there was magic and miracles, there was also messiness and discomfort. Being pregnant and becoming a new parent are among many people's most challenging experiences. I bore witness to the physical discomforts my students experienced each trimester, holding space for the emotional ups and downs brought on by hormones and the dawning experience of "Oh my god, I'm about to have a baby!?" I also saw the exhaustion, pain, and drain of new parenthood. I watched as many students broke down in our check-in circles over challenges feeding their babies, sleeping, or dealing with the physical discomfort that came with holding a baby 22 hours of the day. I saw all the sides of pregnancy and parenthood, not just the beautiful, airbrushed versions seen in the media.

Having seen and experienced all of that, my partner and I *still* decided to have a baby, and 9 years after I began teaching prenatal yoga, I became a mama myself. I was lucky to have an easy pregnancy, but I was also fortunate to have years and years of training and understanding of the pregnancy journey that helped normalize my experience, making everything feel less scary and less uncertain. I was so grateful for this because I found once I stepped onto the mat into "regular" yoga classes as a pregnant person, my experience was anything but. In my experience, teachers in regular classes struggled to help me feel safe and comfortable in my body and left me feeling like I had a major injury rather than simply being pregnant.

Walking into yoga classes once I was visibly pregnant would often elicit looks of fear from teachers. When I told teachers I could modify positions for myself, I could see the relief in their faces. But sometimes I wanted to know what my pregnant students experienced when they attended regular classes and said nothing. I found that teachers either completely ignored me or spent way too much time focusing on me, making me feel like I couldn't do anything. Both experiences were disempowering. Had I not come from a background of in-depth knowledge of yoga and the pregnant body, they also could have been really scary. However, I could empathize with how nerve-racking it might be for a teacher to have a pregnant person in class. I realized how important it was to empower all yoga teachers to understand the needs and capabilities of the pregnant body—to improve the experience for themselves and for their students.

What I hope to offer with this book is a general understanding of the changes that will happen during pregnancy and into the postpartum period. I am not a medical professional and so will offer snippets of information as they apply to the scope of a yoga teacher to help you grasp why we might offer a particular pose or when modifications are helpful. But what I hope you'll take away is more than a textbook accounting of the perinatal period. Instead see this handbook as a resource, a support of sorts, to help you navigate what your students may bring with them to your classes.

PART I

TEACHING
PRENATAL YOGA

CHAPTER 1

Why is Yoga for Pregnant Bodies So Important?

According to a 2016 Yoga Journal study, nearly 75% of yoga practitioners identify as women, and while this statistic excludes transgender folk or non-binary people, given the sheer number, it's likely that at some point—really at many points—one of your students will become pregnant. For those who choose to become pregnant, it's a natural part of a body's life cycle. Yet in the yoga world, pregnancy is often treated as an injury or a special circumstance rather than a norm.

As a teacher, maybe you've had the experience of having a pregnant student take your class. You may have wondered how to best serve them as a student and what was even safe to offer them. As yoga teachers, whether we prepare our classes in advance or teach to the group that walks into the studio, we must always be thoughtful in how we approach the specific needs of our students. And yet often, whether they know it or not, teachers lose students because of their inability to offer adequate support during the pregnancy and postpartum period.

With growing evidence of the health benefits of yoga for pregnant and postpartum students, more and more people are turning to yoga during this important time. Yoga is one of the few things that is consistently recommended by care providers to their students regardless of their experience with yoga prior to pregnancy. As a result, people are searching out prenatal yoga classes, but in areas where there may not be any available, they may be showing up in regular classes looking for support.

Still very few teachers have any training in how to best support these students. Pregnant students are looking for teachers with knowledge and training in how to best provide safe and supportive modifications based on the changes happening in the body during pregnancy. And following pregnancy, students continue to look to teachers for additional support. Many changes that happen during pregnancy—and later, once baby is born—affect the body in the postpartum period.

Indeed, there are very special things about the pregnant body that change the practice of yoga at different points during pregnancy. And our responsibility as teachers is to educate ourselves so we can offer safe and supportive modifications during a period of our students' lives that is a normal part of the life cycle for so many. It's time we stop treating pregnancy as an injury or special situation and recognize the normalcy of pregnancy and our need as teachers to be able to provide support for pregnancy students. The more we as teachers know how to adjust for and support our students, the more our students can not only reap the benefits of yoga during the perinatal period, but also feel strong and powerful in their changing bodies.

Also keep in mind that while many students begin their journey of yoga with prenatal yoga, many are regular and long-time yoga practitioners. There is a deep well of knowledge that comes through the tradition of yoga. For many students, pregnancy isn't a time to put their practice on hold, they will simply need support in adjusting the asana portion of their practice while using the gifts and tools of the other eight limbs of yoga to continue their own growth and potentially navigate all the changes that pregnancy offers. This is why I offer these insights and suggestions for modification within existing practices with the pregnant body in mind. It's not about doing a whole new practice, its simply about taking the wisdom that is already there and ensuring its safe for our pregnant students.

CHAPTER 2

Modifying a Regular Practice for Pregnancy

While many teachers will go on to focus specifically on pregnancy and postpartum practices, a large majority of teachers will find that pregnant students will show up in their regular classes, leaving teachers wondering how to best serve them and what is even safe to offer them. As yoga teachers, whether we prepare our classes in advance or teach to the group of students who walk into the studio, we have to always be thoughtful in how we approach the specific needs of our students. And yet often, whether teachers know it or not, they lose students because of their inability to support them during their pregnancy and the postpartum period.

Pregnant students are looking for teachers with knowledge and training in how to best provide safe, supportive modifications based on the changes happening in the body during pregnancy. And with growing evidence of the health benefits of yoga for pregnant and postpartum students, more pregnant people are turning to yoga during this important time. Still, very few teachers know how to integrate the needs of a pregnant student into their class of non-pregnant students.

If we've planned a specific class, it can feel overwhelming to have a pregnant student join unexpectedly. We may feel concerned that what we've designed will not be suitable for their body. Depending on what you've planned, your comfort level with changing it or offering modifications, and how far along the student is in their pregnancy, you'll have one of three options:

Let the Student Take Care of Themselves

Fundamentally, the goal of this book is to help avoid this. Our goal as teachers should be to teach to whomever enters the room and adjust accordingly. Particularly with something like pregnancy which is a common enough occurrence (unlike, for example, a very specific injury) that teachers should be equipped to respond.

Whether we are new to offering support to pregnant bodies or we simply don't have the bandwidth that day, we teachers can still take steps to make that person a little safer and more confident. At the very least, before class we can run through the list of Poses to Avoid from Chapter 3 with the student or students to give them general guidelines to be aware of. You might also take a moment to demo for them the difference between an open and closed twist.

Clearly, this is the minimal amount of support we want to provide to a pregnant student in our class, but it's certainly better than simply ignoring them.

Offer Modifications and Adjustments

Part of this offering will hinge on how comfortable that student feels about being singled out in class. Some students appreciate the one-on-one attention, as it helps them feel safe, but others—particularly those early in their pregnancy who might not yet be sharing it broadly—may feel incredibly uncomfortable. This is why a conversation before class can help ensure you're meeting a student where they are with a practice that honors not only their pregnant body, but also their mental and emotional state.

Offering individual modifications and adjustments is helpful for teachers who have difficulty pivoting from a planned lesson plan. It allows us to continue with what we planned to offer while ensuring we address the specific physical needs of the pregnant student in our class. It's a convenient option if we're teaching a class style that is inherently less supportive to a pregnant body, such as a vigorous flow class.

You'll find Modifications by Trimester listed in Chapter 3 for each of the major Poses to Avoid to help you assess how best to modify based on your class plan and where the student is in their pregnancy.

Change Your Teaching Plan

Changing your plan can be challenging for those of us who spend time preparing a thoughtful class plan complete with readings or thematic sequences. It can feel challenging and overwhelming to let go of that, but it truly can help us grow as teachers. And this doesn't mean throwing out our whole teaching plan. It often means knowing when to change your teaching plan and when you can offer modifications to pieces you want to retain. Here are some examples of what that might look like:

- Removing or shortening long sequences on the back or offering a bolster to lift the hips for someone in their second or third trimester so they can be on their back longer.
- Limiting the amount of traditional Sun Salutation transitions and flows involving Chaturanga.
- Removing core sequences or offering core work from hands and knees and plank that are safer for pregnancy. (Or offer the pregnant student something else to do during this time.)
- Offer transitions to step to the back of the mat as opposed to stepping forward.
- Limit the number of ups and downs in class. Once you get folks standing, keep them in standing poses for a longer period of time.
- Avoid deep back-bending poses or give options.
- Avoid deep closed twists or give options of open twists.
- Avoid extended periods on the belly or give pregnant students options, whether it's through propping with a bolster or other poses they can do while the rest of the class is on their bellies.

Changing your teaching plan to accommodate the pregnant body is important for so many reasons. First, the more pregnancy friendly your class is, the less you must split your attention by checking in with the pregnant person in the room. You can teach to the whole class rather than just one person. You can know that what you're offering is better suited to their body and you won't have to spend as much time visually checking in to make sure they're okay or that they need modifications.

This also keeps the pregnant person in the room from being singled out. Trust me, they already get it enough throughout the day from people asking them about their pregnancy, making comments about their body, or even unexpectedly touching them. It can be nice for them to feel that they are just another student in the room.

And your non-pregnant students might get to try something new. Classes that are modified to the pregnant body aren't without challenge. Students might move in ways they're not used to, which can be good for everyone. Pregnancy-friendly doesn't mean easy, it just means different. Plus, pregnancy-friendly classes are great for lots of bodies, not just pregnant bodies. Pregnancy specific modifications can be great for folks who have larger bellies, people dealing with low back pain, or folks who have issues with doing tons of Sun salutations.

Finally, you'll grow as a teacher by getting out of your comfort zone and expanding your capacity to adjust and teach to whoever shows up in the room. This benefits you and your students. It's an opportunity to get creative with modifications or alternate poses you might offer. For example, you might have planned a series that included Bow Pose. You can still offer Bow Pose, but you can also have folks roll to their side and take the top heel toward the seat, catching hold of the foot (like in Dancer Pose) and work the opening from there rather than on the belly.

Regardless of what option you choose, it's important to ask all of the following questions when someone walks in your class and shares their pregnancy with you:

- *What's your name?*: This can be helpful if you'll be calling out adjustments or modifications, so you're not saying for the "pregnant person in the room." It also may help them feel a little less singled out.
- *How far along are you?*: This will give you a good idea of what types of modifications they may need based on the trimester they're in.
    - *Do you feel comfortable being on your belly?:* This is a good follow-up question for anyone in their first trimester.
- *Is there anything I need to know about your pregnancy that care providers have mentioned?* And *is there anything specific going on in your body today that is bothering you or needs your attention?*
    - These last two questions can help you figure out any particular things to address or avoid with them.

How To Modify Sun Salutations

A flow class that moves quickly through Sun Salutations is one of the hardest to modify. Here are two ways you can modify Sun Salutations to support pregnant bodies in a regular yoga class:

The first modification for Sun Salutations is more appropriate for the second and early third trimesters, as long as students aren't feeling low back pain when doing unsupported Upward Dogs.

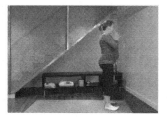

Start in Mountain Pose, as arms are circled out and up, heel toe the feet out to the width of the mat.

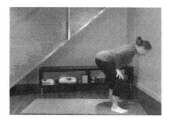

Soften the knees and lower down by sliding the hands down the legs.

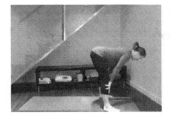

Straighten the legs while coming down and push the shins away to lengthen the legs before sliding all the way to the floor.

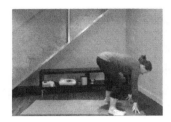

Walk the hands down to the floor, bending knees, if appropriate.

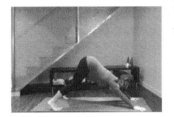

Walk or step the feet back to Downward Dog. Consider keeping the feet wide to support the belly in Downward Dog.

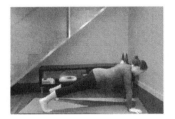

Hug baby toward spine and flow forward into a Plank Pose. Option to hold with the knees lifted or dropped to the floor.

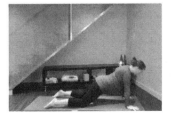

Students will either lower their knees immediately or before moving to Upward Facing Dog.

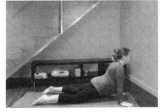

From knees down, allow the hips to lower to find Upward Facing Dog on the knees. Core should be gently engaged through a sensation of "hugging baby toward spine."

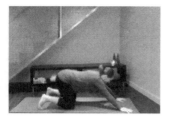

From Upward Facing Dog, keep the knees down, tuck the toes, and glide back through Table Top. From Table Top, hug baby toward spine and lift the hips up and back for Downward Dog.

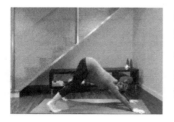

Students can widen their stance to accommodate baby and may find a mat-width distance between feet to be more appropriate. If students are holding here for several breaths, pedaling feet or swaying hips can help address the calf and hip tightness common in pregnancy.

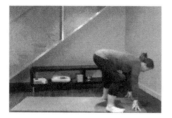

From Downward Dog, keep the feet about mat width apart and step them forward to the front of the mat (this may take several steps). Keep the knees bent to support the back.

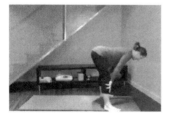

Once at the top of the mat, lengthen the spine by sliding the hands up the legs, just above the knees. Option to fold back down or hold here.

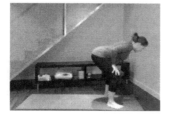

To come to stand, bend the knees, push the hands into the thighs, and lift the spine up to standing.

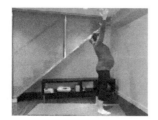

From standing, circle the arms wide and return them to the heart center. Stop here or begin another cycle.

This second Sun Salutation variation is appropriate for all levels of pregnancy and requires the use of a bolster for support.

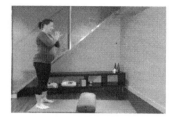

Begin in Tadasana at the back of the mat with a bolster placed about midway up the mat.

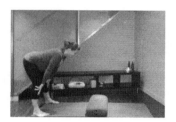

Widen stance to the edge of the mat and slide the hands down the legs to fold forward. Option to add a half lift.

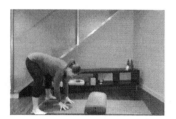

Slide the hands all the way down to the floor and walk them forward.

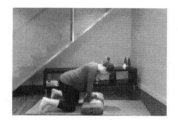

Lower the knees to the mat and walk the hands forward onto the bolster. Continue to walk the hands toward the top of the mat.

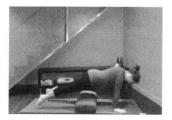

Once hands are at the top of the mat for Plank Pose, tuck the toes and extend the legs. Hug baby toward the spine to support the low back.

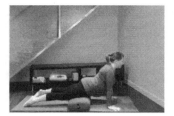

Lower the tops of the thighs to the bolster. The bolster should land below the belly and above the knees to give optimal support for the back and belly in Upward Facing Dog.

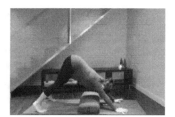

Tuck the toes, lift the hips, and come up to Downward Dog.

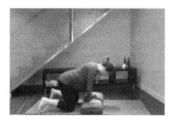

Lower the knees to the mat and walk the hands back to the bolster.

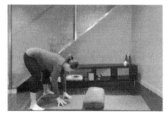

Tuck the toes and lift the hips as the hands are walked back to the feet. Make sure the feet are wide enough accommodate baby.

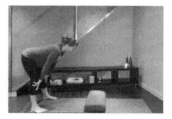

Option to walk the hands up the legs to lengthen the spine and fold forward again. Soften the knees and walk the hands up the legs to come to stand.

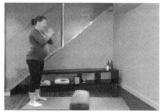

Circle the arms when coming to stand, and end with the hands at the heart center in Tadasana.

CHAPTER 3

Poses to Avoid and How to Modify

Depending on our comfort level with offering modifications, we teachers either can choose to adjust what we're teaching or offer students a general list of poses to avoid to keep them safe. Do note that the more you learn, the more you'll realize that several of the poses in the Poses to Avoid category can be practiced by a pregnant student, they just need to be avoided or modified during portions of their pregnancy.

If a pregnant student shows up in class and you don't have the ability to offer modifications or give them one-on-one attention, you at least can offer them this general list of things to avoid:

Poses to Avoid

- Deep twists
- Poses on the stomach
- Poses on the back where both hips and shoulders are touching the floor
- Deep backbends
- Core work
- Any pose where trauma to the abdomen is a potential risk such as arm balances where the elbow could slip from the hip to the belly.

As you become more skillful as a teacher, the opportunity will arise for you to step in to offer modifications for poses that aren't considered safe for pregnancy and, beyond that, modifications that *are* safe for the student's specific trimester of pregnancy. If you are uncertain of where a student is in their pregnancy, always opt for third-trimester modifications, as that will keep most bodies the safest in poses.

If you have a student asking about a pose that you feel is questionable for a pregnant body, it's important to ask what they're hoping to get out of this pose. It can be hard for some students to let go of parts of their practice, or there might be an ego-based need to prove their body can still perform the same way it did before pregnancy. Help students as much as possible find avenues to still challenge themselves—and perhaps achieve the same goal as the original pose—while keeping them safe. Another question I sometimes ask when someone feels strongly about doing a pose from their prior practice when there's a safer alternative available is, "Do you think this something you can put aside for nine months?" Reminding folks that pregnancy isn't forever and that there are reasons something might be considered less safe can help them make a more informed decision.

Also keep in mind that the first and third trimesters, the pregnancy is considered more at risk. The first trimester because there is a higher rate of pregnancy loss, and third trimester because different factors can contribute to an early birth of the baby. Once pregnancies are in their second trimester they are considered to be a little more stable and this often why students will return to class or join a prenatal class in the second trimester. With this in mind, we want to be mindful particularly around the first trimester. It is never time for students to try something new or to explore things that might be considered questionable. At all times, but particularly the first trimester, erring on the side of caution is always best.

Modifying Twists

When teachers aren't familiar with how to modify their classes for pregnant bodies, one of the many things they will tell pregnant students is that they should never do twists. While this generalization can keep a few folks who shouldn't be twisting safe, for the most part, pregnant folks *can* twist. The twists just need to be modified to suit their bodies, with an awareness of how twists can impact the pregnant body during different trimesters.

FIRST TRIMESTER TWIST MODIFICATIONS

For most folks in the first trimester, twisting is something they can continue to do as long as it feels good for their bodies and there has been no concern with pregnancy loss. The focus during first trimester is on recognizing the increase in relaxin in the body and the intrabdominal pressure that deep twists cause. Initially, students might consider removing deep twists that compress the belly or involve binding.

To modify twists or binds in seated and standing poses, make a little space for the belly rather than finding the deepest version:

- For example, in Marichyasana III, rather than hooking the elbow outside the knee or binding the arms, hold the bent knee with the hand of the arm that would normally hook.

SECOND TRIMESTER TWIST MODIFICATIONS

The second trimester is when baby will start taking up a lot more space in the abdominal cavity. The belly will start to protrude, which makes tight, closed twists impossible. Now is the time to create lots of space for the belly in twists.

To modify twisted lunges and standing twists:
- Consider taking open twists instead of closed twists, such as Side Angle instead of a Lunge with a twist or Revolved Triangle.
- Widen the hand on the ground out to the opposite edge of the mat from the front foot.

To modify seated poses:
- In a pose like Marichyasana III, widen the foot of the bent leg away from the extended leg to make more room for the belly while twisting toward the bent knee.
- Consider taking open twists instead of closed twists, rotating away from the bent leg.

To modify supine twists:
- Try open twists from the chest rather than closed twists from the belly. Start from a side-lying position and open the top arm back and behind so the twist comes from the upper body rather than the lower body. Consider a block or bolster between the knees for better support for the low back.

THIRD TRIMESTER TWIST MODIFICATIONS

At this point, most twists will be relegated to the upper body in poses like Prasarita Padottanasana or in the hips while supine. These twist options will make the most room for baby. They're great options for other trimesters, too, if a student doesn't feel comfortable with a deeper twist at any point in their pregnancy.

To modify twisting on the back:
- Start on the back with knees together feet wide, arms extended out at a T. Drop both knees to one side, to the other.

To modify twisting while standing:
- Take open twists. Twist away from the front leg so the belly remains open. Side Angle will be the best option, with the knee up or down to take the twist in the opposite direction.
  - Offer the option to rest the forearm on the front leg rather than bringing the hand all the way to the floor.

Modifying Poses on the Stomach

For folks beyond their first trimester, staying off the belly feels intuitive, but many will find they will feel fine being on their bellies up till around 14-18 weeks. Others may find immediately that they will feel protective of their belly and want to avoid any poses on the stomach. It's always wise, even if a student is in their first trimester, for teachers to ask if they feel comfortable being on their belly; if they say no, give them options for second and third trimester modifications.

FIRST TRIMESTER MODIFICATIONS FOR POSES ON THE STOMACH

If students feel comfortable being on their stomachs, it is perfectly fine to continue to practice poses that put gentle pressure on the stomach. For most of the first trimester, the uterus is resting behind the pubic bone, which makes gentle pressure on the stomach okay. Poses like Cobra are perfectly fine to continue at this time, though students should consider discontinuing poses that involve work on the belly combined with deep backbending, such as Bow Pose.

If there is concern about being on the belly, sometimes placing a folded blanket underneath the tops of the thighs for poses like Cobra is sufficient relief. Otherwise, folks can swap Cobra for poses that give the belly more space, such as Sphinx and Upward Facing Dog.

SECOND TRIMESTER MODIFICATIONS FOR POSES ON THE STOMACH

Once folks hit the second trimester, being on their bellies will no longer feel comfortable, so teachers will need to modify poses to keep the belly off the floor.

To modify poses like Cobra Pose:
- Consider Upward Facing Dog or Sphinx Pose with a folded blanket placed underneath the tops of the student's thighs.
- Offer Upward Facing Dog with a bolster under the thighs to avoid deep backbending and give support to the low back.

To modify poses like Bow Pose:
- Offer a Single-leg Quad Stretch, either lying on the side or standing to get access to the quads and the chest opener without being on the belly.
- Consider ways that you can move poses that are on the belly to the side or even the back. For example, Bow Pose could become a Quad Stretch or a Bridge Pose.

THIRD TRIMESTER MODIFICATIONS FOR POSES ON THE STOMACH

The modifications for the second trimester listed above still apply, though by the third trimester, some students will find even Upward Dog supported with a bolster too intense.

To modify poses like Cobra or Upward Dog:

- Offer Sphinx Pose with a bolster placed underneath the thighs.
- Flow Cat/Cow while other students are on their stomachs.
- Stay in Child's Pose while other students are on their stomachs.

Modifying Poses on the Back

This becomes an important consideration around 18-20 weeks of pregnancy as baby really starts to grow. When lying flat on the back, baby could potentially put pressure on the vena cava, a vein that carries deoxygenated blood back to the heart. For some people, prolonged pressure on the vena cava can decrease the amount of oxygen to baby and put them at risk.

Keep in mind, it is *prolonged pressure* we are worried about. If a student comes on to the back for a short period of time, they won't do any harm to the fetus. In fact, studies have shown that even when pregnant folks spend extended time on their backs, nausea or dizziness will trigger them to roll over. Students would have to ignore their bodies' extreme cues to remain in an unsafe position on their backs for extended periods of time. That being said, as yoga teachers, we should always err on the side of caution for our students' health and offer safe variations.

FIRST TRIMESTER MODIFICATIONS FOR BEING ON THE BACK

No need to modify being on the back during first trimester. As long as they're at ease, have students take advantage of this time while they can still be safe and comfortable on their backs.

SECOND TRIMESTER MODIFICATIONS FOR BEING ON THE BACK

Around 18-20 weeks, the main thing for students to modify will be Savasana and extended periods on the back.

To modify Savasana:

- Use a bolster underneath the length of the spine or set up in any of the more supported Relaxation Poses for Savasana, which are safe for students throughout all three trimesters. (See options in Chapter 7)

To modify extended time on the back:

- Invite them to roll to the side between poses or come up to a sit if they notice nausea, dizziness, or lightheadedness during extended time on the back while doing leg or hip work.

THIRD TRIMESTER MODIFICATIONS FOR BEING ON THE BACK

At this point, most students will likely feel uncomfortable lying flat on their backs for any extended period.

To modify leg work on the back:

- Place a bolster or folded blanket underneath the hips and lift the hips up off the floor.
  - If this feels uncomfortable (and it may for students late in third trimester, as it will push baby's weight toward their lungs and stomach), they can also do leg work in the Reclining Relaxation Pose.

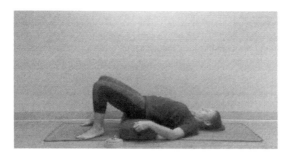

To find support for lift of hips for poses on the back, have students begin in Bridge Pose. When they lift the hips, they will slide a bolster or a blanket folded to a least 2 inches of thickness under their hips.

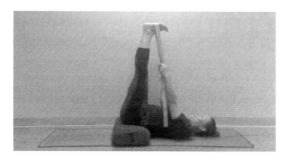

In poses like Viparita Karani or Supta Padangusthasana, use the lift under the hips. A strap around the feet will also allow them to hold for a longer period of time.

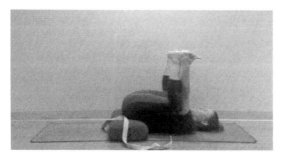

Happy Baby Pose can also be supported with a bolster or folded blanket.

Modifying Deep Backbends

Backbending poses are difficult for the body later in pregnancy and should be gradually adjusted for over the course of nine months. The issue around backbending is because of several things:

1. Most pregnant folks toward mid to late second trimester are already spending the majority of their day in a backbend, so there's no need to take the spine further into this shape.

2. Backbends lengthen the linea alba, the connective tissue running at the midline of the rectus abdominis. Extra stretch on the linea alba can potentially exacerbate diastasis recti.

3. As baby gets bigger, pregnant students lose the core support necessary to bring them in and out of deep backbends and can injure low back muscles being overloaded by deep backbends.

FIRST TRIMESTER MODIFICATION FOR BACKBENDING

At this point, the main modification will be to avoid deep backbends on the belly like Bow pose. Other than that, if deep backbends are a regular part of someone's practice and they continue to feel good doing those poses, they can consider continuing. The main thing to keep in mind is the levels of relaxin in the body rising over the course of each week and the body's tendency to overstretch ligaments and tendons (which is a lot more common in big poses). Students will want to have an awareness to not push right up to the edge of their flexibility.

SECOND TRIMESTER MODIFICATIONS FOR BACKBENDING

As students move into the second trimester, and particularly toward the end, teachers should offer adjustments to provide support. Toward the middle and end of the second trimester, as baby grows, the belly will start stretching. We'll want to be wary of adding strain on the linea alba. At this time, back muscles will also start doing more work to support posture and, therefore, will need more support in backbending poses to get in and out.

Consider having students back off their backbends, adding support as needed:

- Use a block under the hands in Camel Pose if they were used to bringing the hands to the heels. Or have them bring their hands to their low back and keep them there instead of going all the way toward the heels.
- Transition from doing Wheel Pose to Bridge Pose.
- Focus more on a quad stretch for Dancer Pose as opposed to the backbend.
- Consider dropping the knees to the floor for Upward Facing Dog.

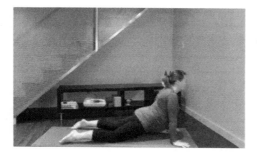

Upward Facing Dog with the support of knees down.

THIRD TRIMESTER MODIFICATIONS FOR BACKBENDING

Once students are in their third trimester, it will most likely feel uncomfortable to do any kind of deep backbending, or they may find that getting out of a deep backbend will be difficult. Now is the time to offer further support in backbends. Additionally, this is when these movements will be the most likely culprits to contribute to diastasis recti postpartum. While diastasis can be triggered by doing core work, it can also be made worse by stretching the linea alba.

To give support for backbends in third trimester:
- Offer a bolster under the thighs for Upward Facing Dog.
- Avoid deeper backbends or backbends that require core engagement to get out of like Camel Pose.

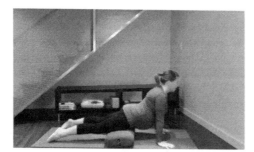

For Upward Facing Dog, set the bolster at the top of the thighs, just below the belly but above the knees to provide optimal support for low back and belly.

Modifications for Core Work

Core work is super tricky in terms of what pregnant students can and can't do. Students, in general, think they must avoid core work altogether, but there is a lot of functional core-based work they can do that will help them retain some abdominal support which, in turn, will also support the low back.

But the hard part is students who want to push doing core work through their pregnancy, due in large part to the pressure on new parents to "bounce" back postpartum. As a result, some folks feel added pressure to start strengthening their core while they're still pregnant in preparation.

We teachers should support our pregnant students' goal of maintaining a strong core, in terms of the obliques and transverse supporting the back in holding baby's weight. But we should caution against abdominal strengthening exercises like sit-ups, crunches, and Boat pose that can make diastasis recti worse.

FIRST TRIMESTER MODIFICATIONS TO CORE WORK

At this point, it's still okay to do a lot of asana requiring core. The reason we avoid core work, for the most part, is the strain it puts on the linea alba, combined with the load put on the rectus abdominis during core-based movements that can make diastasis recti more likely or worse. In the first trimester, baby is quite small, so the belly generally is not getting drastically larger, to the extent that it would put load on the connective tissues and muscles. The main thing to avoid is anything that puts the belly in deep compression (think sit-ups and crunches). Otherwise, students can continue to do poses like Boat Pose and Plank Pose if they feel comfortable.

SECOND TRIMESTER MODIFICATIONS TO CORE WORK

Once students are halfway through the second trimester, usually around 18-20 weeks, they will start to notice more substantial growth of the belly. They may even experience the sensation of the belly stretching or baby getting bigger. Once this begins, it will be time to remove core work from the practice entirely, particularly Boat Pose or specific core work sequences on the back. That doesn't mean that pregnant students can't work their core; it will just look different.

Core work for the pregnant body looks more like using the weight of the belly as a counterweight to engage support muscles like the obliques and the transverse abdominals. In any pose where a student might have hugged their belly in prior to their pregnancy, they can now do the same on the cue to "hug baby in." This action of hugging baby in can help engage the obliques and deep transverse. By hugging baby in toward the spine in the following poses, folks can do core work during a sequence or poses in class that otherwise are no longer appropriate for them:
- Opposite Limb Extension with arm and leg lifts
- Hydrant Lifts
- Plank Pose (on or off the knees)

THIRD TRIMESTER MODIFICATIONS TO CORE WORK

Now is the time for students to be extra mindful of their core. They'll want to ensure they do the following:

- Avoid traditional core work and practice the options listed in second trimester modifications.
- Roll over to their side to come up or down from lying on the floor.
- Modify or discontinue poses where they can visibly see doming happen at the midline of the abdomen.
- Avoid anything that triggers a burning sensation at the midline of the abdomen. This is a sign that there is pulling or stretching of the linea alba.

Poses Where Trauma to the Belly is Possible

For the most part, yoga is low impact and so trauma to the belly is not generally a possibility. That being said, several arm balance poses require the support of elbows very close to the abdomen and slipping could potentially cause trauma. Students should avoid poses like this immediately and throughout the duration of their pregnancy. If there is ever a question of the possibility of injury or trauma to the abdominal region, avoid the pose. Remind them its only for the next 9 months.

Other Things to Avoid in Yoga

- Certain Pranayama: Kapalabhati, Bhastrika, long breath retentions
- Kriyas: Uddiyana Bhanda, Nauli, Agni Sara
- Hot Yoga

Certain Pranayama and Kriya

There are certain Pranayama and Kriya that we want students to avoid during pregnancy either because of the pressure they put on the belly or because of the risk of depriving the body of oxygen. The Pranayama practices to avoid include: Kapalabhati, Bhastrika, and long breath retentions. The Kriyas to avoid are: Uddiyana Bhanda, Nauli, and Agni Sara.

MODIFYING PRANAYAMA FOR ALL TRIMESTERS

The right pranayama practices can be excellent during pregnancy to help relieve stress. They also can help students practice connecting to their breath as a tool during labor. Instead of the practices above, consider offering these options (find out more about these practices in Chapter 8):

- Equal inhale/equal exhale breath
- Lengthening the exhale in relation to the inhale

- Villoma Pranayama
- Nadhi Shodhana Pranayama

Hot Yoga

It bears mentioning here since many students may be practicing hot yoga prior to their pregnancy that hot yoga classes should be discontinued as soon as students know they are pregnant and avoided for the duration of their pregnancy. The reasons behind this are threefold:

- Body Temperature: most importantly is the potential for a hot yoga practice to increase the internal temperature of the pregnant person's body. Significant body temperature increases during pregnancy put the fetus at risk and should be avoided.
- Over-Stretching: the added heat in a hot yoga class combined with relaxin in the body makes the possibility of overstretching muscles, tendons, and ligaments—possibly causing injury—much more likely.
- Lightheadedness, Dizziness, Shortness of Breath: all these common side effects of pregnancy can be made worse by heat and are another reason hot yoga should be avoided.

CHAPTER 4

The Role of a Prenatal Teacher & Prenatal Yoga Class

For many people the practice of yoga has been transformative during difficult times physically and emotionally, and many people find a sense of deep community within their yoga classes and at their studios. Prenatal classes will most likely offer both these things for yoga students. As prenatal yoga teachers, we hold a special space for students in their lifetime. Pregnancy marks a time of profound change for people both personally and in the greater scope of their relationships, families and even their jobs.

Pregnancy is also a time of huge change physically which can bring its own sense of challenges, but also an opportunity to connect with the deep wonder of the miraculous capacity of the body. As teachers, we not only hold the deep well of wisdom of the yoga practice, but we also hold the spectrum of the experience of pregnancy and we hold it again and again as we welcome new students to our classes.

Prenatal yoga classes and the role of a prenatal yoga teacher are unique to this population of students and as a result, there are several things for us to keep in mind.

Your Role as a Prenatal Yoga Teacher

One of the key pieces to prenatal yoga is the importance of remembering your scope. It may feel like we need to know everything about pregnancy, yoga and birth. However, our role as a yoga teacher is to know how to guide students through yoga poses that are safe for the pregnant body. Students have care providers to teach them about everything else.

Your Scope as a Yoga Teacher

It is not your job nor is it in your scope of practice to offer medical advice or to question a care provider's recommendation. Always refer students to their care provider for advice that is out of your scope. If you're offering suggestions in circle, encourage them to ask their provider first before trying something.

If a student is feeling uncertain, scared, or worried about what a care provider has told them, do encourage them to seek out a second opinion and let them know that no matter how far along they are in their pregnancy, they can switch providers to find a better fit.

- This is particularly important for pregnant students of color and students with larger body types, who often do not receive the same level of support regarding complications and issues with their pregnancy. You can be their advocate to help them find the support they need.

Do be an advocate for students if they feel uncertain or worried or if they need resources. Have a list on hand of providers that you know and trust. I recommend having one or two of the following folks in each category to recommend:

- Acupuncturist
- Doula
- Chiropractor
- Massage therapist
- Physical therapist (at least one who specializes in pelvic floor health)
- **And** if you want to broaden your level of support:
  - Perinatal mood disorder support (often your state will have a 1-800 number)
  - Pregnancy loss support
  - Childbirth educator
  - Lactation specialist
  - Postpartum doula

Setting up the Yoga Space

If possible, practicing in a circle can be hugely beneficial for pregnant students for several reasons:

- They can then set their mats up at the wall and use the wall for support in certain poses.
- It facilitates the energy of the circle and creates a sense of connection and community with other people in the room.
- It can also help give them visual feedback of what a pregnant body looks like in a pose. Even though you may be demoing, students might find it helpful to look around the room at other pregnant students to see how their bodies might look in a pose.

If possible, every student should have a blanket, bolster, and two blocks. If you are teaching in a studio without props, consider encouraging students to bring a blanket from home. At the very least, a blanket can help provide padding for achy joints and a lift for seated positions to make the back and pelvis more comfortable.

Because of the impact of hormones on the body, pregnant folks will often feel heightened senses, which can cause them to feel nauseous, overwhelmed, or overstimulated more easily in their environment. Consider the following:

- Smell: Most pregnant folks, especially in the first trimester, will be extra-sensitive to smells. Try to ensure the studio environment is as scent-free as possible. This includes avoiding incense and aromatherapy and also airing out the space if a previous class was particularly sweaty.
- Sound: Music can make it easier for students to focus and stay aware of their physical bodies, but be mindful of volume, as sounds may seem extra-loud or distracting to pregnant folks. If you use music in your classes, be mindful of your choices; consider softer instrumental music rather than music with vocals. (But avoid instrumental tracks with the sound of water. Pregnant folks already have to pee a lot as it is!)
- Temperature: In general, pregnant folks will run a little hotter than non-pregnant students. Keep studio temperatures a couple of degrees cooler. If the class before you warmed up the room, try airing it out to keep the room slightly cooler.
- Unsure about any of these? Always encourage your students' feedback about the room and their comfort level.

The Role of A Prenatal Yoga Class

Prenatal yoga classes offer an experience and community that is unique to the period of pregnancy. Students can still attend "regular" yoga classes but may find that they don't get all of the same benefits that prenatal classes provide.

Give Students the Opportunity to Connect with Their Own Bodies

One of the important pieces the prenatal yoga practice can teach students is the wisdom inherent in their own bodies. It can teach them how to feel more comfortable moving in their own bodies and listening to feedback their bodies may give them about what is and isn't working. This is extremely important as they approach childbirth and can be an invaluable tool for navigating labor and postpartum.

Our goal as prenatal teachers is not to make sure that every student looks perfect in a pose or that their alignment is exactly right. It's more about ensuring they are safe in the pose and adjusting the shape of the pose to suit their body that day and as their body changes from trimester to trimester. (Triangle Pose at 12 weeks is very different from Triangle at 38 weeks!) With that in mind, keep adjustments to a minimum. However, if students are in alignment that could cause injury or discomfort, provide them adjustments to keep them safe.

If you are someone who likes to give hands-on adjustments, consider giving adjustments that will help them feel some relief from common pregnancy discomforts and always ask for consent before touching anyone:

- Pressure upward on the iliac crest during Downward Dog can help lengthen the low back, providing low back relief.
- Pressure on the outer hips/gluteus medius in Right Angle at the Wall or Prasarita Padottanasana can provide low back relief.
- Pressure on the sacrum moving toward the tailbone in Child's Pose can provide low back relief.

Encourage Students to Listen to Their Own Bodies

- Give them the option to take breaks and rest if they feel dizzy, nauseous, light-headed, or tired. The first time you offer them Child's Pose can be a good place to mention that this is a good pose for them to come back to if they need that break.
- Encourage students to use the restroom whenever they need to, as pregnant folks will be more likely to need it during class.
- Encourage water breaks during class so students can stay hydrated. They're great when students are transitioning up and down from the floor.
- Some students will need to snack during class if they deal with low blood sugar or nausea. While it's not often encouraged in yoga spaces, make sure students know it's okay to bring snacks to their mat with them.

Allow Students to Connect with the Experience of Being Pregnant

It is my personal opinion that a great deal of focus is put on the baby over the pregnant person, even during pregnancy. Pregnant folks often feel like they are merely a vehicle for baby, rather than an incredibly powerful, strong person growing another human being. Wow! This focus on baby before they even arrive often translates into postpartum, when the new parent becomes lost in the experience and will sometimes put off taking care of their needs—medically, personally, and emotionally—in order to take care of baby.

Let your yoga classes be an opportunity for students to focus on themselves so they can set up this healthy relationship to the self as they move through their pregnancy and into parenthood.

Help them explore their changing body during pregnancy. This can work two ways:

- Invite them to stay present in the process, as it will go by quickly (even if it doesn't feel like it at the time).
- Encourage them to also know that if things are hard or uncomfortable, they will change, whether it's throughout their pregnancy or once their pregnancy ends.

Some folks may like the opportunity to connect with baby. Here are some ways to encourage connection with baby that don't feel overbearing or forced:

- If you're incorporating something like flowing arms in and out of a Warrior II or a squat position, offer them the option to bring their hands to their belly.
- During Meditation or Pranayama practice when there is focus on the breath, remind them that they are not only breathing for themselves but also for baby.
- When opening or closing practice, rather than Anjali Mudra, offer one hand on heart, one hand on belly.

Validate the changes that students experience in their bodies throughout their pregnancy:

- In balance poses, remind them how balance shifts as baby grows and they might notice a change in their balance from week to week.
- Acknowledge that they will need increasing room for baby as baby grows in poses like Child's Pose and Downward Dog. Always give them the option to explore wider stances.
- Encourage them to observe changes they notice when doing their check-in circle. It can also be helpful for students to hear that others are also experiencing the same changes—physically, mentally, and emotionally—that pregnancy can bring.

Acknowledge that the changes aren't just physical and they're continuous. Students will find their relationship to being pregnant, approaching childbirth, and being a new parent will change through the course of their pregnancy, and they might experience a myriad of different emotions about each stage. Reassure them that worry, fear, anxiety, and stress are all valid feelings.

Creating Inclusive Prenatal Yoga Spaces

Prenatal yoga classes are inherently inclusive and exclusive at the same time. There is an overarching connection among students around the shared experience of pregnancy, however the variations of experiences and also identities and backgrounds of students make that experience incredibly different. Our role as a yoga teacher in this space is recognizing the broad range of experiences for our pregnant students and working to make our classes and our language as inclusive as possible.

Teach to the Range of Students Present

This is where a check-in circle can be so helpful. For example, simply knowing that the majority of your students are in their third trimester versus their first trimester might change how quickly you cue each move or the poses you offer.

The check-in circle can also give you clues to particular pregnancy discomforts that your students are experiencing so you can offer poses to alleviate those discomforts or provide cues about movements to avoid that might trigger those things.

Be Mindful About How You Speak About Birth in Your Classes

Birth and the choices that people make around it are very different and specific to their own needs, circumstances, and pregnancies. Ensure that your language around birth is supportive of all choices:

- Use the term provider instead of midwife or doctor.
- Use the term unmedicated birth instead of natural birth.
    - Talk about coping during labor without talking badly about medical interventions and C-sections. Some people make choices for medication or C-sections prior to birth and for some folks, the need arises, despite their plans otherwise, during the birth process. It is not our role as yoga teachers to promote one kind of birth plan over another; that is a student's private decision. Our goal is to help students feel at ease and peace with their plans for birth and avoid creating shame or blame around their choices.

Be Inclusive of All Experiences

Be mindful about using words like father, dad, and husband. Not everyone has a male partner, not everyone is married to their partner, and some people are single parents either by choice or circumstance.

- Use the term partner or even birth partner to be inclusive if you're talking about support during birth.

Not all pregnant folks identify as women, ladies, gals, etc. Try to keep language as inclusive as possible around gender.

- When addressing the class use terms like you all, y'all, everyone, and all of us. You also can use students' individual names, since you'll learn them in circle.
- When talking about pregnancy and birth use words such as pregnant folks, pregnant people, pregnant students, birthing folks, birthing people.
- When talking about after baby arrives use the terms parent and parenthood.

Some people love being pregnant. Some people hate being pregnant. Some are excited about having a baby, and some are scared. Remember that when speaking about the experience of pregnancy, childbirth, and parenthood.

CHAPTER 5

The Circle

. I recommend beginning each class with an opening circle. An opening circle can be long or short, depending on how many people are in the room and how in-depth you want to go with students. Even if you are pressed for time or have a large group, holding a quick circle to check in with students will benefit you and them in the following ways:

- It gives you an opportunity to introduce yourself, share your background, and establish a relationship with students.
- Students can build community through shared experiences. Simply in learning each other's names they're more likely to connect with one another after class.
- It gives the you the opportunity to find out what is going on with bodies in the room so you can offer sequencing, poses, and options to address these aches and pains or to avoid certain issues.
- You also can create community by opening up the circle to questions and recommendations, allowing other students to be the experts and provide advice to their fellow students.

If you anticipate folks will be sitting for some time, though, offer them different poses or props that can make them more comfortable in their seat. For example, if you have a large group of students and you know the circle will cut into time you had planned for asana, consider offering them different seated asanas to do while in the circle and pausing every so often to have them switch.

Questions to Ask in Circle

- What's their name?
- How many weeks along are they?
- Is there anything you should know about from their care provider?

Additional Questions to Ask

- Anything that they want to focus on today that's tired, sore, or tight?
- Is there a pose that they do or don't want to do today?
- How is their energy level today? Thumbs up? Thumbs down? Or neutral?
- What pronouns do they use?
- Is there anything they want you to know today about how they're feeling?

Questions to Ask to Start Discussions

- Is anybody having trouble sleeping? Any tips that are helping them get a little more sleep?
- Anyone dealing with swelling in their feet? What's working for them?
- It's really hot today. How are they dealing with the heat?
- What kind of support are they considering during labor?
- Ask the group for recommendations of providers folks like: massage therapists, acupuncturists, physical therapists, childbirth educators, doulas. Pick one and highlight the benefits of working with that kind of provider.

Things NOT to Ask in Circle:

- When is their due date?: This makes it hard for you to calculate how many weeks pregnant they are (unless you're super amazing at fast math), and it reinforces the expectation that the due date is important. Babies are so rarely born on their due dates that helping students let go of the focus on the due date can be helpful.
- Have they been pregnant before/How many kids do they have?: Folks may share this in circle, but focusing on it by asking is a potential trigger for those who have had trouble conceiving or experienced pregnancy loss.

Holding Space in Circle

Depending on how much time you allow for discussion, circles can sometimes bring up tough issues, even if we try to keep them super simple. But being prepared to handle difficult or uncomfortable situations can make you feel a little more at ease.

Discomforts & Complaints that Appear Serious

The following are potentially signs of pre-term labor and if a student mentions any of them in circle or at any point during class, encourage them to discontinue what they're doing and contact a care provider immediately:

- Vaginal bleeding

- Regular painful contractions
- Amniotic fluid leakage

Things You Don't Know

If a student brings up something you don't know about—for example, a particular diagnosis from a doctor or issue you're unfamiliar with—that's okay! Here's how to handle it:

- Acknowledge that is new to you and ask them what their provider has told them about the issue.
- Ask them if they were told of anything they should or shouldn't be doing, with regards to their yoga practice.
- Let them know you'll do some research so you can better understand their experience and prepare for the next class.
- Let other folks be the expert. It can be empowering for other students—and help foster community—for other folks to offer answers to questions or provide recommendations. If it feels appropriate, you can easily open it up with, "Has anyone dealt with this? What worked for you?" Just be ready to step in if other students provide inaccurate information. Otherwise, let them support one another. This is also helpful if you don't have any ideas or recommendations.

Inclusive Language

If someone is using language about themselves or someone else that is not inclusive, take the time to offer language that is inclusive and why. This can build community by ensuring everyone feels their individual experiences are represented and respected. It may even encourage contributions from students who may not have spoken up otherwise.

Challenging Situations & Feelings

If a student is having a hard time, validate whatever they are feeling. If they're unhappy or not enjoying something, reassure them that those feelings are okay and that everyone has different experiences during pregnancy.

- If someone has a more loaded or specific issue going on, offer to connect with them after class to provide more detailed recommendations or support.

CHAPTER 6

Creating a Prenatal Yoga Class

When teachers begin creating classes for prenatal students, they might feel intimidated and overwhelmed. There's an added level of anxiety in teaching to pregnant students that something a teacher offers may cause injury or harm. We might also simply worry about the difference in working with the pregnant population. There are a few simple things to consider when planning a class and some things to keep in mind about pregnant students. But just like any other yoga class, your prenatal classes will be taught to students with a range of abilities in their bodies, potential body discomforts, and differing levels of experience with yoga.

Putting together prenatal sequences can feel daunting for new teachers, but this book gives you a good introduction to poses, movements, and mindsets that can be healing and restorative for your pregnant students. Teachers often feel they must offer individual and unique sequences for each class. That is 100% not necessary, in general, but also for several reasons specific to a prenatal class:

- *Flexibility*: Your classes will ideally focus on the specific needs of the bodies in the room, so keeping your planned sequence flexible will be a great benefit to your students.
- *New students*: Because pregnancy only lasts about nine months, you'll only have your students with you as pregnant people for a short period of time. Even if students start their prenatal practice with you early in their pregnancy, they'll only be with you for around seven months at the most. You'll constantly have new students who have never practiced prenatal yoga—or simply yoga while pregnant—with you before.
- *Simplicity*: "Pregnancy brain" is really a thing. Students will often complain of their brain feeling foggy and not having as good of a memory before they got pregnant. Students will be less likely to remember week to week what you offered in previous classes.
- *Confidence*: Because their bodies are changing so rapidly, students might appreciate the opportunity that doing the same pose week to week gives them to:

o   Create a sense of safety in poses that are familiar to them, even though their body may feel different. They will only have to navigate how their body feels in the pose class to class, not how to do unfamiliar poses each time.

o   Have the space to actually notice that their body has changed and feels different.

o   Explore their changing balance in poses as baby grows.

Creating Prenatal Yoga Class Sequences

Sequencing a prenatal yoga class can look very similar to a regular yoga class, but given there are certain needs for pregnant bodies, there are a few things to keep in mind as you create prenatal seuqnces.

Avoid a Lot of Ups and Downs

Because pregnant folks tend to have lower blood pressure and higher heart rates, there is a tendency to become lightheaded, short of breath, and dizzy—not to mention that the bigger baby gets, the harder it is to get up from the floor and get back down again. For these reasons, we try to avoid moving up and down from the floor too much in a prenatal class. In general, start students out on the floor with seated and warm up poses, bring them to standing for standing and wall poses, then bring them back down again for seated and floor poses before Savasana.

Be Aware of Circulation in Long Holds

Because of lower blood pressure, students will have slower blood circulation, so it is important to stay aware of long holds in poses as students' extremities may begin to tingle and become numb much more quickly than they might have prior to pregnancy.

- For seated poses that might be held for a long time, like Virasana, give students the option to come out if they start to feel uncomfortable. If they do need to come out, show them other ways they might sit comfortably.

- For standing poses that you are planning to hold for a while, like Warrior II, consider offering an option to flow in and out of the pose.

- Notice that in poses where the arms are overhead, like Warrior I or Chair Pose, fingers will much more easily go numb. Offer arm flows or the possibility of bringing the arms out of the pose but staying with the position of the legs.

Use Neutral Poses to Balance and Contain

Because of relaxin in the body, it can be easier for the pelvic joints to move out of alignment, particularly when we spend a lot of time on one side of the body doing a series of poses. Because we put pressure on the front and back of the pelvis (at the pubic joints and SI joints), we want to help bring the pelvis back to neutral after spending time on single-sided poses.

For example, after doing a sequence of Warrior I to Warrior II to Triangle Pose on one side, teachers should pause in a neutral pose before repeating on the other side, and then again before returning to the initial side. If you know that you have students in the room dealing with significant issues like SI joint pain or pubic symphysis, provide the option to add a block between the thighs in the neutral pose with some squeezes to help enhance the containment and help further invite the pelvis back to neutral. Here's what neutral poses might look like throughout a class:

- Warm-up poses: Cat/Cow, Child's Pose, or Downward Dog
- Standing poses: Chair Pose and Squats
- Wall poses: Right Angle or Chair Pose at the wall
- Seated poses: any of the symmetrical seated poses like Bound Angle or Wide Angle
- Floor poses: Bridge Pose

Be Aware of Overstretching of Muscles and Ligaments

Due to the relaxin that starts flooding the body soon after pregnancy begins, muscles and ligaments are more vulnerable to overstretching than in non-pregnant bodies. A good measurement for students to think about is stretching at about 85% of their capacity. Pregnancy isn't the time to be pushing to the extreme of a stretch, especially if folks notice they have more mobility, as it becomes a lot easier to go too far.

To help protect students from overstretching:
- Avoid extremely long, deep stretches.
- For longer stretches, set them up with props to better support their bodies.
- Notice hyper-mobile folks (this is generally easiest seen in folks who tend to hyperextend in elbows or knees) and offer them alignment cues around keeping a micro-bend to joints even in poses where the limb is "supposed" to be straight.

Keep It Simple

As mentioned above, don't worry about complicated flows and new classes every time you teach. Keep your sequences and your cues simple and straightforward. Pregnant folks often come to class with all sorts of things going on mentally about their pregnancy, approaching birth, or parenthood. Mentally they might not be as present, and all the hormones in their bodies have been shown to impact clarity of thought. Keep your cues short and direct about where you want them to go and what you want them to do or focus on. Then when you've got them in the pose, if you want to get more into alignment or talking about the benefits of a position, spend some time talking about it once their bodies are already there.

The Flow of a Prenatal Yoga Class

As you create a sequence for prenatal classes, sometimes it will depend on the energy of the room, sometimes it will depend on the weather and temperature of the room, and sometimes it will depend on the time of day. Here are a few class outlines you can use to put together a 75-minute class:

MORNING CLASS

Opening circle: 10 minutes

Seated poses with Pranayama or meditation: 10 minutes

Warm-up poses: 15 minutes

Standing poses: 20 minutes

Wall poses: 10 minutes

Floor poses: 5 minutes

Relaxation: 5 minutes

EVENING CLASS

Opening circle: 10 minutes

Warm-up poses: 10 minutes

Standing poses: 25 minutes

Wall poses: 10 minutes

Seated poses: 10 minutes

Relaxation with Pranayama or meditation: 10 minutes

LOW-ENERGY/HOT DAY CLASS

Opening circle: 10 minutes

Floor poses: 15 minutes

Warm-up poses: 15 minutes

Seated poses: 15 minutes

Legs Up the Wall variations: 10 minutes

Relaxation with Pranayama or meditation: 10 minutes

HIGH-ENERGY CLASS

Opening circle: 10 minutes

Warm-up poses: 15 minutes

Standing poses: 25 minutes

Wall poses: 10 minutes

Seated poses: 5 minutes

Relaxation: 10 minutes

Prenatal Yoga Sequences

As you begin teaching, creating entire sequences can feel daunting. The following sequences are meant to provide inspiration. You may find you teach the whole sequence pose by pose or take these sequences as framework to start building your own. You'll find in the following chapter in-depth descriptions of the poses listed below.

A Basic Prenatal Sequence

Opening Circle

Warm Up

- Seated side stretch and neck stretches
- Cat/Cow
- Child's Pose
- Do this series on one side, and repeat on second side:
    o Opposite Limb Extension
    o Gate Pose
    o Lunge
    o Downward Dog

Standing

- Chair Pose with block between thighs
- Do this series on one side, and repeat on second side:
    o Warrior I
    o Warrior II
    o Exalted Warrior
    o Extended Side Angle
    o Squat

Balance/Wall Poses

- Tree Pose
- Right Angle at the wall
- Low Squat with Pelvic Floor work

Seated

- Wide Angle with side stretches and fold
- Bound Angle

Floor

- Clamshells
- Bridge Pose

Savsasana

A Sequence for Tight Legs

Opening Circle

Seated

- Seated side stretch and neck stretches
- Sama Vritti Pranayama practice

Warm Up

- Cat/Cow
- Child's Pose
- Do this series on one side, and repeat on second side:
    - Opposite Limb Extension
    - Shoulder/Neck Release
    - Lunge
    - Ardha Hanumanasana
    - Downward Dog

Standing

- Chair Pose with block between thighs
- Do this series on one side, and repeat on second side:
    - Warrior I
    - Warrior II
    - Triangle Pose
    - Squat

Balance/Wall Poses

- Chair Pose at the wall
- Quad Stretch
- Right Angle at the wall
- Low Squat with Pelvic Floor work

Seated

- Janu Sirsasana
- Bound Angle

Savsasana

A Sequence for Hips

Opening Circle

Floor

- Do this series on one side, and repeat on second side
  - Side-lying outer leg work
  - Side-lying inner leg work
  - Bridge Pose

Warm Up

- Cat/Cow
- Child's Pose
- Do this series on one side, and repeat on second side:
  - Hydrants
  - Vasisthasana
  - Hip Flexor Release
  - Gate Pose with hands on the floor and hip circles
  - Downward Dog

Standing

- Chair Pose with block between thighs
- Do this series on one side, and repeat on second side:
  - Warrior I
  - Warrior II
  - Side Angle Pose
  - Wide Legged Forward Fold (with twist on first side)

Balance/Wall Poses

- High Squat
- Hip Stretch at the wall
- Right Angle at the wall
- Low Squat with Pelvic Floor work

Seated/Floor

- Pigeon Pose
- Bound Angle

Savsasana

A Sequence for Preparing for Labor

Opening Circle

Seated

- Seated Pose with neck stretches
- Meditation for Preparing for Birth

Warm Up

- Cat/Cow
- Child's Pose
- Do this series on one side, and repeat on second side:
  - Hydrant Lifts
  - Gate Pose
  - Lunge
  - Gate Pose with hands on the floor and hip circles
  - Downward Dog

Standing

- Chair Pose with block between thighs
- Do this series on one side, and repeat on second side:
  - Warrior I
  - Warrior II
  - Squat
- Chair Pose with block between thighs

Balance/Wall Poses

- High Squat
- Tree Pose
- Right Angle at the wall
- Chair Pose at the wall
- Low Squat with Pelvic Floor work

Floor

- Bridge Pose
- Supine Twist

Savsasana

A Sequence for Low Energy

Opening Circle

Seated

- Seated Pose with neck stretches
- Seated Wide Angle with side stretches and fold

Warm Up

- Cat/Cow
- Child's Pose
- Do this series on one side, and repeat on second side:
  - Opposite Limb Extension
  - Neck/Shoulder Release
  - Lunge
  - Hip-Flexor Release
  - Child's Pose
- Downward Dog

Balance/Wall Poses

- High Squat
- Tree Pose
- Right Angle at the wall
- Low Squat with Pelvic Floor work

Seated

- Bound Angle
- Forward Fold

Floor

- Bridge Pose
- Side-lying Outer Leg Work
- Side-lying Inner Leg Work
- Supine Twist

Savsasana

- Legs up the Wall (with different leg variations)
- Stay or transition to a different Savasana shape

A Sequence for Back Pain

Opening Circle

Warm Up

- Cat/Cow with flow back
- Child's Pose
- One Arm Dog
- Do this series on one side, and repeat on second side:
  - Opposite Limb Extension
  - Neck/shoulder release
  - Lunge
  - Downward Dog

Standing

- Chair Pose with block between thighs
- Do this series on one side, and repeat on second side:
  - Warrior I
  - Warrior II
  - Exalted Warrior
  - Extended Side Angle
  - Wide Angle Forward Fold (with twist on first round)

Balance/Wall Poses

- Quad Stretch
- Right Angle at the wall
- Pelvic Rocks at the wall
- Low Squat with Pelvic Floor work

Seated

- Wide Angle with side stretches and fold
- Seated Pose with neck and chest release
- Forward Fold

Floor

- Bridge Pose
- Supine Twist

Savsasana

CHAPTER 7

Prenatal Yoga Poses

The poses outlined here are certainly not an exhaustive list of yoga poses. They are, however, poses that will be safe for the majority of bodies throughout the longest period of time during pregnancy and that will provide support or relief for some of the common discomforts that arise during pregnancy. Pregnancy-related issues and discomforts may make these poses less comfortable or less viable in the body, but, for the most part, most students will be able to explore these poses.

The poses are broken down into sections in a way that may make it easier to then create yoga sequences, though seated and floor poses may also be done at the beginning of class before or after warm-up poses, depending on the sequencing of the class.

The descriptions presume a familiarity with the poses and provide cues that may be more appropriate or specific to the pregnant body. You'll also find benefits and contraindications listed for the poses. Use the poses and sequencing tips from Chapter 6 to create your own prenatal yoga sequences.

Warm-up Poses

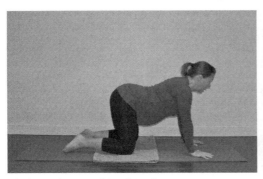 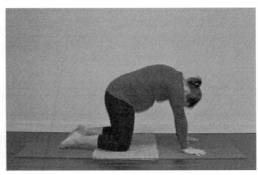

Chakravakasana (Cat/Cow)

Start from Table Top, with knees under hips and hands under shoulders.

Avoid a large curve of the low back in Cow and exaggerate the spine in Cat Pose.

When coming into Cat, hug baby in toward the spine, push the floor away, and arch the back toward the ceiling.

Flow in and out of these two poses or add a flow back to Child's Pose from Cat (be sure to widen the knees).

Benefits: addresses low back tightness and pain.

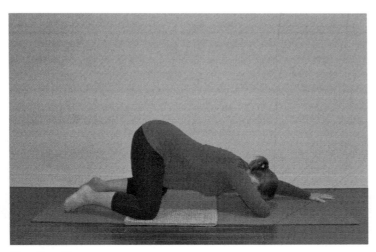

One Arm Dog

Begin in Table Top, drop one arm with the forearm parallel to the front of the mat, just in front of the fingertips of the other hand.

Walk the other hand forward and lower the forehead to that first forearm. Ensure that hips stay over knees.

Hug baby in toward the spine to support low back.

Benefits: releases mid/upper back, shoulder, and neck tension.

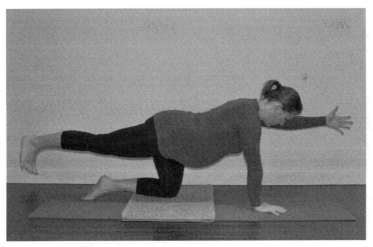

Opposite Limb Extension

Begin in Table Top and extend one leg back with toes on the floor.

Push into the hands and hug baby toward the spine, then lift the leg.

Once leg is lifted, option to add the opposite arm.

Can add flows of the arm and leg raising and lowering for more strength building.

Benefits: pregnancy-appropriate core and low back strengthening.

Contraindications: SI joint pain (keep foot on floor), modify for wrist issues.

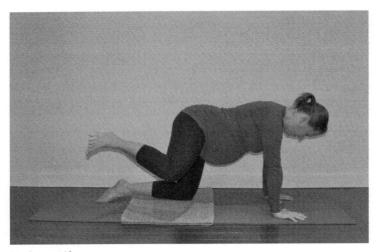

Hydrant Lifts

Start in Table Top and open one knee out to the side. Keep lifting leg bent, with knee at 90 degrees.

It is not about how high the leg is lifted, but about keeping the hips level.

Raise and lower the leg within comfortable range of motion for hip and low back.

Benefits: opens and strengthens tight or weak hips.

Contraindications: SI joint pain (keep knee low to floor), pubic symphysis.

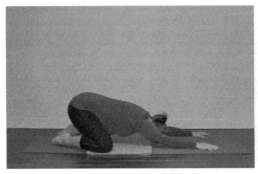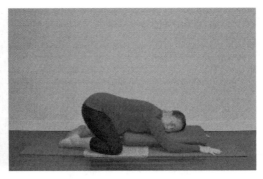

Balasana (Child's Pose)

Begin in Table Top, widen knees to accommodate baby's size and bring big toes to touch.

Sit weight back toward the heels as far as knees or hips allow.

If arms overhead is uncomfortable, stack palms or fists under forehead.

Can do supported option with a bolster set under the head and chest to allow space for baby.

Benefits: releases low back tension.

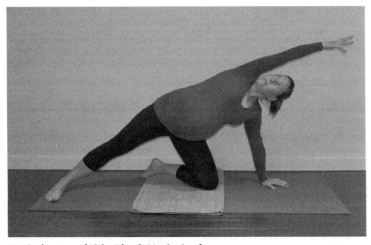

Vasisthasana (Side Plank Variation)

Begin in Opposite Limb Extension with the toes of the extended leg on the floor.

Pivot the heel of the extended leg to the floor and circle the same side arm up toward the ceiling and eventually alongside the ear. Kick foot of bent knee back as far as needed for support of balance.

Option to reach top arm to ceiling, circle behind back for neck release, or lift the extended leg for hip strengthening.

Benefits: opens side body and offers core strengthening appropriate for pregnancy.

Contraindications: modify for wrist issues.

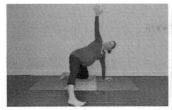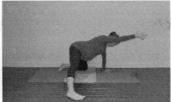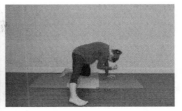

Shoulder/Neck Release

Begin in Opposite Limb Extension with the back toes up or down, move leg to the side with leg hovering or toes dragging on the floor.

Place foot parallel to the long edge of the mat, inner arch in-line with inside of bent knee.

With hands under shoulders, lift the arm of the extended leg side and hold.

Move to flow after the hold, encourage students to alter movement as it feels good for them.

Benefits: releases neck or shoulder tension, opens pelvis. *Contraindications:* pubic symphysis.

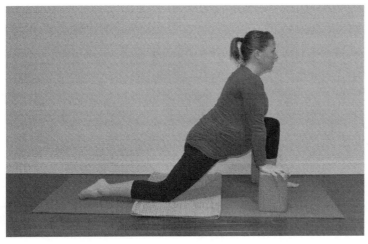

Low Lunge

Transition to this pose is often done from one leg extended out to the side. From there, heel-toe foot forward bringing it just to the inner edge of the mat.

Front foot should be near the edge of the mat to allow room for baby.

Option to use blocks (both inside front foot) or lift arms up to higher version.

Benefits: releases tight hip flexors, creates space in pelvis.

Contraindications: SI joint pain, pubic symphysis.

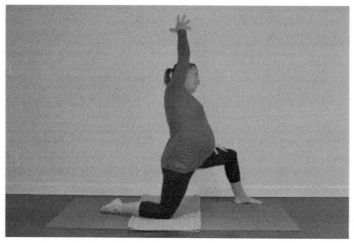

Low Lunge + Hip Flexor Release

Begin in Low Lunge with arms at the sides, ensuring hips are over back knee.

Drop tailbone and lift pubic bone to activate hip flexor.

Lift arm of back leg side and tip up and over toward bent knee side.

Benefits: releases tight hip flexors.

Contraindications: SI joint pain, pubic symphysis.

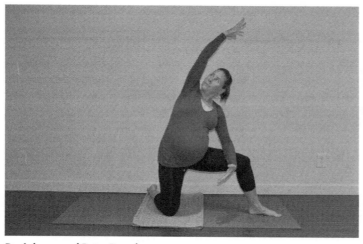

Parighasana (Gate Pose)

Standing foot in alignment with inner knee of knee down.

Option to reach top arm to ceiling or circle behind back for neck release.

Lower hands to floor and do hip circles to release hips.

Benefits: open side body, create space in pelvis.

Contraindications: pubic symphysis.

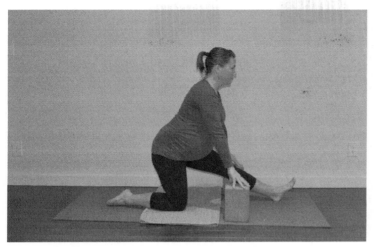

Ardha Hanumanasana

Transition to this pose is often done from one leg extended out to the side, from there heel-toe foot forward bringing it just to the inner edge of the mat.

Front foot kept wider than traditional pose to allow room for baby.

Sit the hips back and slide the front leg heel forward to extend the forward leg. Flex the foot and draw the toes toward the body. Both blocks may be kept inside front leg.

Benefits: releases tight hamstrings.

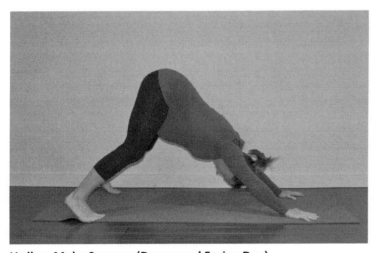

Urdhva Muka Svanasa (Downward Facing Dog)

Begin in Table Top, tuck the toes and lift the hips up and back.

Practice with feet at least hip-width apart, perhaps even as wide as the mat. Hug baby up and in toward spine to support low back.

Knees may need to be bent to lift hips up and back to take the weight off of hands and wrists.

Benefits: moves baby's weight out of pelvis, stretches calves, lengthens neck.

Contraindications: carpal tunnel, swollen hands, headaches, heartburn.

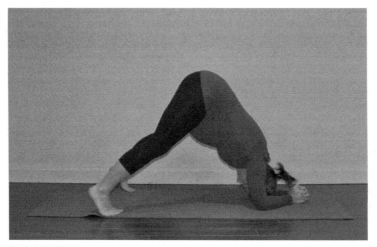

Dolphin Pose

Begin in Table Top, lower the forearms to the floor with the elbows where the palms just were.

Ensure elbows are no wider than shoulder width apart.

Interlace the fingers to create a stable base and tuck the toes and lift the hips up and back.

Just like Downward Dog, practice with feet hip width apart or wider.

Step feet in slightly closer to elbows than stance for Downward Dog.

Bent knees will often make pose more accessible.

Benefits: moves baby's weight out of pelvis, stretches calves, lengthens neck.

Contraindications: headaches, heartburn.

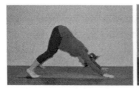 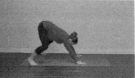 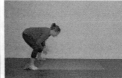 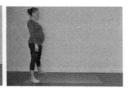

Transition to Standing

If a student has chosen Dolphin Pose, have them briefly change to Downward Dog to make coming to stand easier.

From Downward Dog, widen feet and walk hands back to feet.

Option of Forward Fold or high Squat at back of mat, depending on what is comfortable.

From high Squat, brings hands to thighs and press to standing.

Contraindications: dizziness, lightheadedness (come up slow, come up on exhale).

Standing Poses

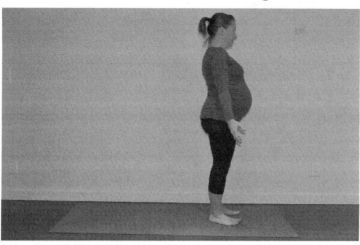

Tadasana (Mountain Pose)

Stand with feet at least hip-width apart, even wider if there is hip pain.

Watch for students locking their knees.

Benefits: grounds and stabilizes.

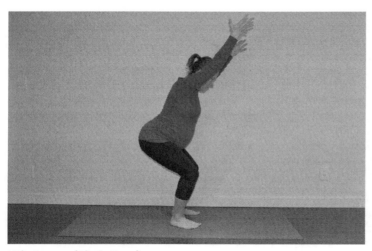

Utkatasana (Chair Pose)

Begin in Mountain Pose and bend the knees, inviting the weight to move back into the heels.

Ensure the knees are tracking toward second toes and not wobbling in or out.

Keep feet hip-width apart to support balance.

Options for arm variations and flowing the arms.

Teach with block between thighs to encourage inner thigh and outer hip strengthening.

Benefits: strengthens legs.

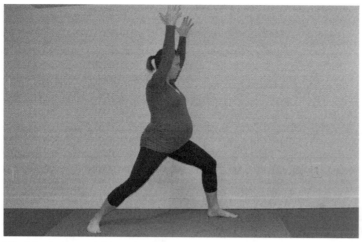

Virabhadrasana I (Warrior I)

Begin in Mountain Pose and step back with one foot, heel-toe it back once or twice to accommodate the width desired between feet.

Widen front foot to the side to support balance.

Bend the front knee over the ankle and extend the arms up alongside the ears.

Benefits: strengthens and lengthens legs.

Contraindications: SI join pain (shorter stance), pubic symphysis (shorter stance).

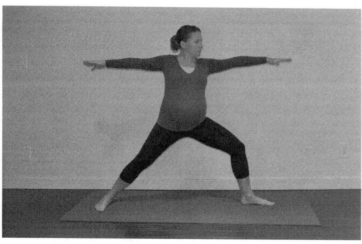

Virabhadrasana II (Warrior II)

From Warrior I, heel-toe wider front foot back in, straighten front leg, and parallel feet.

Heel-toe the back foot back further for the longer stance of Warrior II.

Bend front knee over ankle and extend arms toward the front and back of the mat.

Rather than sinking into the legs, imagine dragging feet toward one another to engage legs.

Benefits: strengthens and lengthens legs, opens hips and pelvis.

Contraindications: sciatica (front leg straight, feet parallel), pubic symphysis (shorter stance).

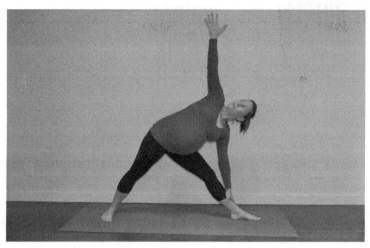

Utthita Trikonasana (Triangle Pose)

From Warrior II, straighten front leg. If stance feels too long, bring the back foot in slightly.

Bring back hand to hip, front hand to thigh.

Slide the front hand down the leg, landing above or below the knee.

Option to extend the top arm or keep the hand on the hip to avoid numbness.

Benefits: strengthens and lengthens legs, opens hips and pelvis.

Contraindications: sciatica (front leg straight, feet parallel), pubic symphysis (shorter stance).

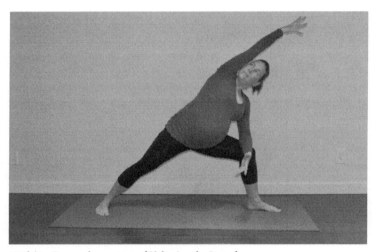

Utthita Parsvakonasana (Side Angle Pose)

Begin in Warrior II and either lower the forearm to the thigh or keep the arm straight and put the hand on thigh.

Bring the back arm up toward the ceiling and then extend along the ear.

Option to add different arm variations to release neck and shoulders.

Benefits: strengthens and lengthens legs, opens hips and pelvis.

Contraindications: sciatica (front leg straight, feet parallel), pubic symphysis (shorter stance).

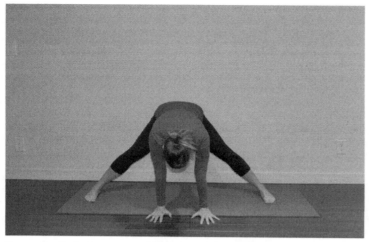

Prasarita Padottanasana (Wide Legged Forward Fold)

From Warrior II, straighten the front leg and parallel the feet.

Ensure both feet are on the same parallel line.

Come forward by sliding hands down the legs to prevent low back strain.

Can offer many variations, hands under shoulders, twist, Downward Dog arm position.

Benefits: moves baby's weight out of pelvis, lengthens legs.

Contraindications: headaches, heartburn (keep head in line with heart).

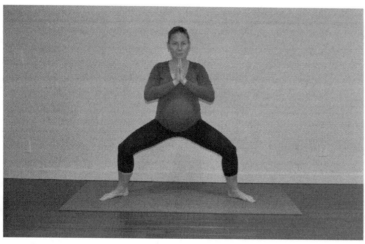

Standing Squat

From Warrior II, straighten the front leg and parallel the feet.

Consider bringing feet closer together if stance feels too wide.

Bend knees and ensure knees don't go past toes. Toes can be turned out or feet parallel.

Options to flow in and out, challenge the legs with a hold, and add arm flows.

Benefits: strengthens legs, opens pelvis.

Contraindications: placenta previa (shallow squat), breech presentation (shallow squat).

Balance Poses

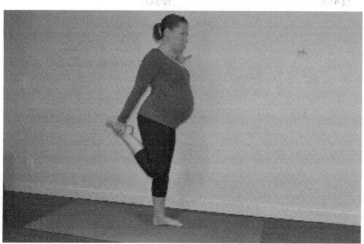

Quad Stretch

Start about 2 feet from the wall, with enough room to touch the wall with elbow bent but still feel some space between the body and the wall.

The inside foot is the standing foot, bend outside leg knee and catch hold of the foot, use a strap if unable to reach foot.

Tilt tailbone down, lift pubic bone to support low back and deepen stretch.

Option to keep inside hand on wall, slide hand up the wall, or move hand away from wall.

Benefits: stretches quadriceps, challenges balance.

Contraindications: SI joint pain (don't do side that hurts).

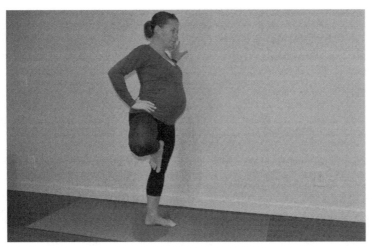

Vrikshasana (Tree Pose)

Start about 2 feet from the wall.

The inside foot is the standing foot. Bring outside foot to inner ankle with toes on the floor.

Option to stay here or slide foot up to inner calf or inner thigh, avoid pressure on side of knee.

Hand can stay on wall, elbow can be kickstand, or can take hands off the wall.

Benefits: strengthens legs, supports changing balance, opens pelvis.

Contraindications: SI joint pain (don't do side that hurts), pubic symphysis (knee forward).

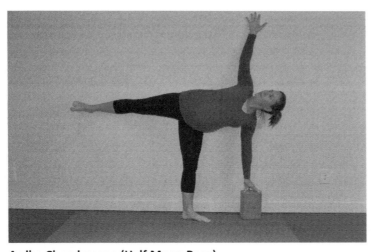

Ardha Chandrasana (Half Moon Pose)

Begin in Triangle Pose with back to the wall and with block on the floor. Bend front knee to reach for block, and place hand on block.

Bring the back against the wall and push into the standing leg, lifting the back leg to come up. Option to not lift top arm.

Benefits: strengthens legs, supports changing balance, opens pelvis.

Contraindications: SI joint pain (don't do side that hurts), pubic symphysis.

Poses with Wall Support

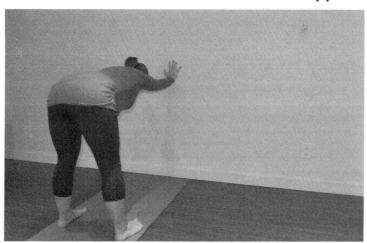

Right Angle at the Wall

Hands start on wall in line with low ribs. Feet step back, at least hip-width apart, to create right angle. Hug baby toward spine to support low back and deepen low back stretch.

Option to add swinging hips or pedaling feet.

Benefits: releases low back.

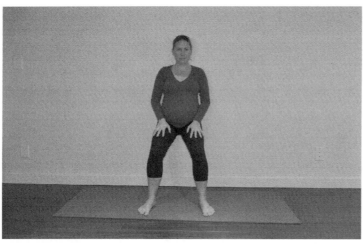

Pelvic Tilts

Bring the back to the wall and walk the feet forward about two feet.

Keep feet at least hip-width apart. Knees can be as bent or straight as student prefers.

Tip tailbone toward wall on inhale, pubic bone toward ceiling on exhale. Movement comes from tipping pelvis not bending and straightening legs.

Benefits: lengthens low back and releases tension.

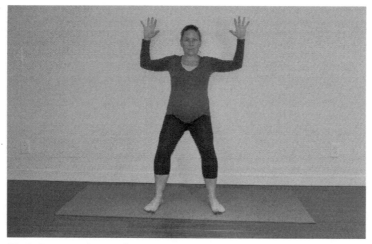

Chair Pose at the Wall

Bring the back to the wall and walk the feet forward about two feet.

Keep feet at least hip-width apart or wider, knees as bent as student prefers.

Options for arm variations: arms straight, elbows, bent, arms down.

Benefits: strengthen legs, a pose to explore the intensity of labor.

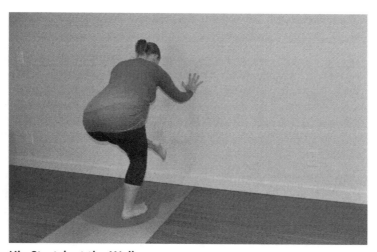

Hip Stretch at the Wall

Begin about 2-3 feet away from wall (hip tightness dictates distance).

Slightly bend standing knee, hook ankle of opposite foot like Thread the Needle, then walk hands down wall.

Sit weight down and back much like in Chair Pose.

Benefits: releases hip tightness, strengthens legs.

Contraindications: SI joint pain (don't do side that hurts), pubic symphysis.

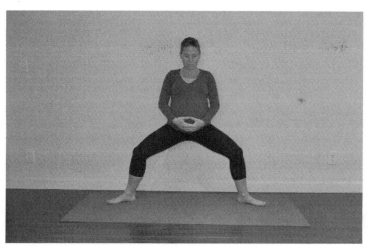

High Squat

Bring the back to the wall and walk the feet forward about one foot.

Heel-toe the feet out to the side, the width of stance depends on depth of squat (do not track knees past ankles).

Explore arm variations.

Benefits: opens pelvis, strengthens legs.

Contraindications: pubic symphysis, a pose to explore the intensity of labor.

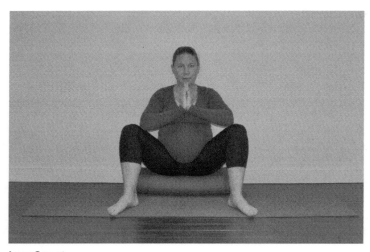

Low Squat

Start standing with feet as wide as the bolster and back against the wall and slide down wall onto a bolster.

Feet may need to move away from the bolster to make room for baby.

Benefits: opens pelvis, creates good place to do pelvic floor work. Good transition to seat.

Contraindications: pubic symphysis.

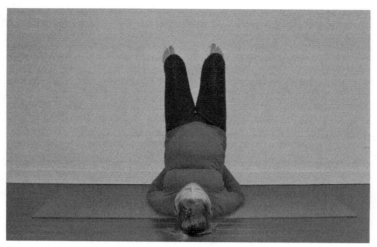

Sarvangasana (Shoulder Stand)

Start in Legs Up the Wall with no lift, hips right against wall.

Knees are bent at 90 degrees and feet push into wall to help lift hips.

Support the low back with hands.

Slide a bolster under back to rest or when ready to come out.

Benefits: relieves weight of baby in pelvis, may help resolve breech presentation.

Seated Poses

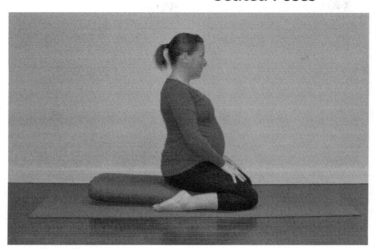

Virasana (Hero's Pose)

Use block or bolster to prop pelvis and blanket to pad and support, keep knees in line with hips.

Tuck blanket under ankles to prevent discomfort in top of foot or ankle.

Options to add neck, wrist, and arm stretches.

Benefits: opens quadriceps, addresses cramping in front of lower legs.

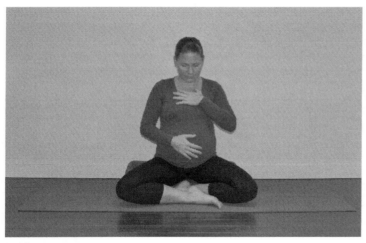

Sukhasana

Always prop with bolster or folded blanket under seat.

Option to add neck stretches, wrist stretches, and shoulder release.

Benefits: creates comfortable seated position for most pregnant bodies.

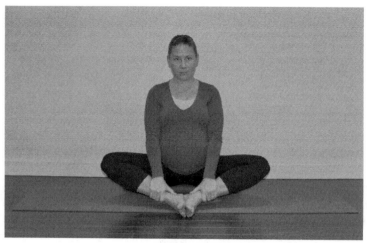

Baddha Konasana (Bound Angle)

Prop with a bolster or folded blanket under seat.

Option to place blocks under knees for those with knee or hip pain.

Option to stay upright or walk hands into forward fold.

Benefits: opens tightness in inner hip and groin.

Contraindications: pubic symphysis.

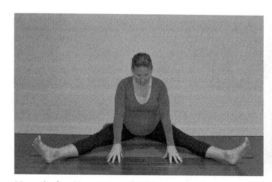
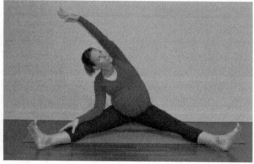

Upavistha Konasana (Wide Legged Seated Forward Fold)

If propping up on bolster, offer rolled blanket or blocks under knees.

Option to include chest opener or forward fold.

Option to add side bend for opening side body and back.

Benefits: opens pelvis, lengthens hamstrings, lengthens side waist.

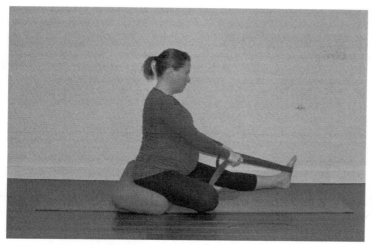

Janu Sirsasana (Head to Knee Forward Bend)

Use a strap to loop the extended leg foot.

Keep spine long, engage foot, and move heart toward toes.

Option to fold over centerline or toward bent knee if baby is inhibiting fold.

Benefits: opens pelvis, lengthens hamstrings.

Contraindications: pubic symphysis.

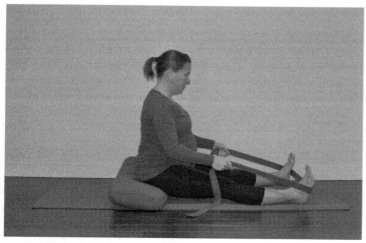

Paschimottanasana (Forward Fold)

Use a strap to loop the feet and give extra stretch to legs.

Rather than folding forward, keep spine long, engage feet, and move heart toward toes.

Keep feet at least hip-width apart (leg angle depends on size of baby).

Benefits: lengthens hamstrings and calves.

Floor Poses

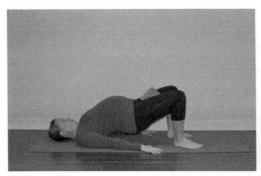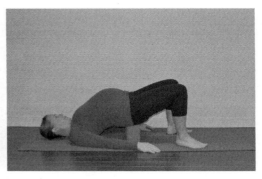

Setu Bandha Sarvangasana (Bridge Pose)

Place block between upper thighs. Set feet hip width apart, with heels under knees.

Push into feet, squeeze block and lift hips away from the floor. Option to flow or hold.

Options to add block squeezes, hip dips, and pelvic floor lifts to strengthen.

Benefits: strengthens glutes, low back, and legs, opens hip flexors.

Contraindications: SI Joint pain (try supported version with block).

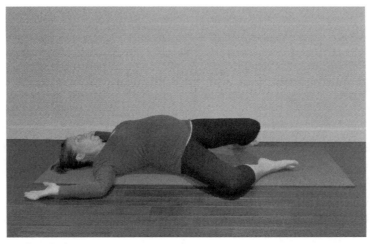

Supine Twist

Start with feet hip-width apart or wider.

Arms reach out a T-shape or with elbows bent depending on shoulders and space in the room.

Let the knees drop to one side and as knees twist one direction, head goes the other.

Benefits: lengthens low back, opens chest.

Contraindications: pubic symphysis, SI joint pain.

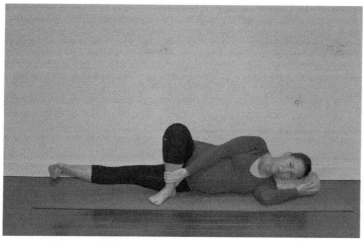

Side-Lying Inner Leg Work

Prop head with folded blanket or bolster.

Bend top leg and place in front of extended bottom leg. Extended bottom leg should be in line with spine and foot flexed and parallel to the floor.

Ensure hips are stacked and level. Raise and lower bottom leg.

Benefits: strengthens inner thigh.

Contraindications: pubic symphysis.

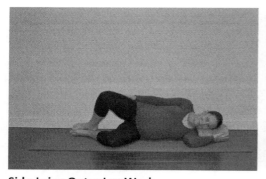
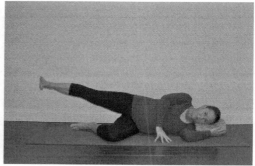

Side-Lying Outer Leg Work

Prop head with folded blanket or bolster.

For clam-shells, knees will be bent and stacked, ankles remain together as top knee lifts and lowers. Ensure hips stay stacked and level.

Option to also extend top leg out, flex foot and parallel inner seam to the floor.

Keep leg extended straight, as if it is an extension of the spine, ensuring the leg doesn't move toward the front or back edge of the mat. Raise the leg only high enough that there is challenge but hips can stay stacked.

In either pose, the top hand can press down on the top leg to increase difficulty.

Benefits: strengthens outer hip. *Contraindications*: pubic symphysis.

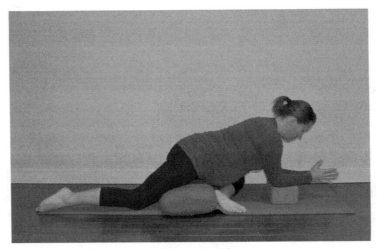

Eka Pada Rajakapotasana (Pigeon Pose)

Start in Table Top with bolster under knees.

Draw one knee forward and pivot at the knee to bring foot forward of bolster.

Slide other knee back off bolster so front of hip is resting on bolster and extend leg.

Angle away from bent knee of forward leg if baby inhibits forward fold.

Support with bolster or block under torso/arms.

Benefits: opens hips. *Contraindications:* sciatica, SI joint pain.

Relaxation Poses/Savasana

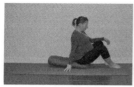 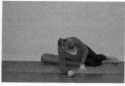 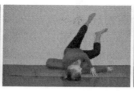 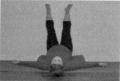

Viparita Karani (Legs Up the Wall)

Place bolster with the long edge against wall.

Sit on the short edge of the bolster with side of body touching the wall.

Bring outside arm to the floor and rotate hips toward the wall so butt is touching it.

Bring head to the floor and scoot closer to the wall.

Use legs and the push off top hand into the floor to help rotate the legs up the wall.

Offer leg variations: legs together, legs wide, bound angle, squat at the wall.

Benefits: addresses swelling of feet and general leg discomfort.

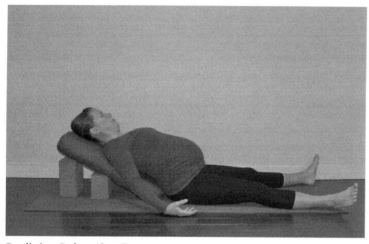

Reclining Relaxation Pose

Use two blocks a few inches apart (one standing vertical behind one standing horizontal) to support reclining bolster.

Offer a folded blanket under seat for low back and tailbone support.

When lying back, ensure that low back is up against the bolster and entire spine is supported by it.

Offer leg variations: knees bent with feet on floor, legs long, bound angle.

Benefits: offers a way to lie on the back that is safe in pregnancy.

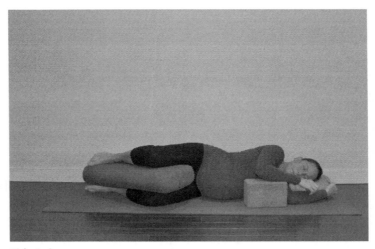

Side Lying

Place folded blanket under the head.

Place bolster between knees or under top bent knee while bottom leg is straight.

Place block under top arm to support overstretching in the back.

Option to place a flat blanket under bottom hip for added padding.

For those in the third trimester, option to tuck a blanket between belly and the floor to give a little lift to belly and prevent baby's weight from pulling on the low back.

Benefits: offers best option for support when lying down for those late in pregnancy or experiencing discomfort in other poses.

CHAPTER 8

Pranayama for Pregnancy

The thing I tell my students about breath is that it is the one thing they will have with them throughout their pregnancy, during labor, and into postpartum. They won't always be able to do a yoga pose—especially while in labor—but they will always be able to breathe. And one of the things students share with me postpartum time and time again is that their ability to connect with their breath helped them during labor. Not remembering a pose we did. Not how I talked about managing labor. It was simply their ability to continue to breathe and connect with their breath that helped them navigate the challenges of labor.

With that in mind, know that Pranayama need not be complicated for prenatal students. In fact, simple is better. As teachers, it's also important for us to be aware of breath length and recognize that many students will have shorter breath cycles as early as their second trimester, so we want to give shorter cues and also give people the option to stop if they feel dizzy or lightheaded.

Sama Vriti

This is one of the simplest Pranayama practices and is generally quite accessible for most pregnant folks. It can help address stress and provide calm and presence. Have students start by finding a comfortable position for their body, whether it is sitting up or lying down. You can also do this practice going into Savasana or coming out of Savasana.

You can take each of the steps from 10 to 20 breath cycles, until students reach the balanced breath, then have them stay there for 2 to 5 minutes.

Guide them through the following steps:

- *Allow the eyes to close half way or all the way, and, if it feels comfortable, bring your hands to rest on your belly.*
- *Start by bringing your attention to your breath. You may start by noticing the breath flowing in and out of the nostrils. Perhaps feeling the sensation of the movement of breath over the top lip. Or you might notice that there's a slight coolness on the inhale and a warmer sensation on the exhale.*
- *Now become aware of your breath by noticing the movement of your belly. As you inhale, direct the breath into your hands letting your belly expand like a balloon filling with air. And as you exhale, let your belly empty, deflating like a balloon emptying of air. Inhale, let the belly expand as fully as possible, and exhale, let the belly empty of breath completely.*
- *Once you have access to this movement of breath, bring your awareness to the inhale and exhale. Start to lengthen and even out the breath. Let your inhalation be as long as your exhalation. You might start by inhaling to a count of four and exhaling to a count of four. Gradually increase the inhale to a five and exhale to a five. Sometimes holding a count of our breath can help our mind stay present and ensure we keep up the balanced inhale to exhale.*
- *When you're ready to release a practice, take a few easy breaths and notice any changes that you feel before you open your eyes.*

Lengthen the Exhalation

This is another simple practice that should be accessible for most students. (You can make it even more accessible by encouraging them to let the exhalation become as long as feels comfortable for them.) This particular Pranayama practice can be helpful for stress and anxiety or as a practice before bed if they have difficulty falling asleep.

Encourage students to find a seat that feels comfortable. Consider offering the wall for support for the back in a seated pose or encouraging them to take a Reclining Relaxation Pose if sitting for an extended period feels uncomfortable. Remind them that with any breath practice during pregnancy there should never be a time when they feel dizzy, lightheaded, or struggling to breathe. If that happens, instruct them to stop the practice immediately.

Guide them through the following steps:

- *Close your eyes if that feels comfortable and start by tuning into your breath. As you inhale and exhale, let your breath gradually lengthen and deepen. This doesn't have to happen immediately; overtime, let it be gradual and without rush. Notice if there are stutters or stops in the breath and see if you can smooth them out.*
- *Now begin to match your inhalation to your exhalation. (In this practice, I'll offer an inhale of 4 and an exhale of 4.) Continue this for approximately 10 rounds of breath or until you feel that the breath is flowing easily and smoothly. Again, this doesn't need to happen immediately, but can happen slowly over time.*
- *Now we'll start to lengthen just the exhalation. In this example, inhale to a count of 4 and now exhale to a count of 5. Repeat this for approximately 20 rounds of breath or until you feel the breath is flowing easily and smoothly.*
- *Now if you feel that the exhalation of breath is right at the edge of your comfort level, stay with this. If you feel that you can lengthen your exhalation further, we will continue, extending the exhalation to a count of 6 or even 7. Continue for approximately 10 rounds of breath until you feel the breath is flowing easily and smoothly.*
- *Once you are ready, release the counted breath and return to an easy breath for a few rounds before opening your eyes.*

Nadi Shodahana (Alternate Nostril Breathing)

Another breath practice that can be helpful for stress and anxiety or to help calm a busy mind.

This breath practice can be done either using the fingers to close off the nostrils or simply by using the direction of the mind to bring focus to breath moving in and out of one particular nostril. This practice is often taught with a certain breath count and breath retentions. For the sake of the different needs of pregnant bodies and the varying breath capacities of students, it can be helpful to get students started with an example but then let them continue on their own so they can use a breath length that works for them.

Have them begin by finding a comfortable seat, they might consider using the wall as support if that will help them sit more comfortably.

Guide them through the following steps:
- *Begin by placing the thumb of the right hand on the right nostril and the ring finger of the right hand on the left nostril. The pointer and mild fingers can either rest gently on the forehead between the brows or curl into the palm.*
- *Begin with the fingers resting lightly so that breath can travel in and out of both nostrils.*
- *Bring the attention to the breath and notice the inhale and exhale of the breath. Take a few breaths inviting the breath to become smoother and longer.*
- *With the next inhalation, close off the right nostril and inhale through the left for a count of 4.*
- *At the top of the inhale, close the left, open the right nostril, and exhale out of the right for a count of 4.*
- *Inhale on the right side, the same side, for a count of 4.*
- *At the top of the inhale, close off the right and open the left and exhale for a count 4. This is one round.*
- *Continue to inhale on the left for a count of 4, close off the left, open the right, and exhale for a count of 4. Inhale the same side for a count of 4, close off the right, open the left, and exhale through the left for a count of 4. This is two rounds.*
- *You will continue through four more rounds on your own. If you find the breath to be too long or too short, you can lengthen the breath or shorten it. If you find you get dizzy or lightheaded, end the practice.*
- *Your final round will end with an exhale out through the left nostril. When you complete this last round, lower the hand, take a few breaths, and notice what you feel.*

Viloma Pranayama

This Pranayama is another breath practice recommended for calming the nervous system. Because this has slight holds and longer extension of the inhalation, it's not recommended for pregnant folks who are already experiencing extreme shortness of breath or lightheadedness.

Encourage students to find a seat that feels comfortable. Consider offering the wall for support for the back in a seated pose. Remind them that with any breath practice during pregnancy there should never be a time when they feel dizzy, lightheaded, or struggling to breathe. If that happens, instruct them to stop the practice immediately.

The focus of this practice will be on the inhalation and breaking it into three parts. The inhalation will remain ongoing and will come in through sips of air until the inhalation is complete. The exhalation will be one long breath out.

Guide them through the following steps:

- *Close your eyes if that feels comfortable and start by noticing your breath. Notice your inhale and exhale and how it moves in and out.*
- *Turn your awareness to your inhalation, and with the next several breath cycles, we will break the breath into three sips of air. If you get lightheaded at any time, stop the practice.*
- *With the next inhalation, take a sip of air, about a third of your breath. Pause. Take another sip, another third, and pause. And then take the final sip of breath, completing your inhalation.*
- *Allow your exhalation to be one smooth long breath out with no stopping of the breath and without letting the breath burst out of the body.*
- *With the next inhalation, go back to sipping in the breath three times, then release one solid exhalation.*
- *Take this practice at your own pace, and let your sips be as long or as short as they need to be. If it feels interesting to you, you can add slightly longer pauses between each sip. Always let your exhalation be one long, fluid breath out.*
- *Complete 10-15 breath cycles, and then return to watching your normal inhale and exhale.*

CHAPTER 9

Meditations for Pregnancy

Pregnancy can be a time of varied emotions, highs and lows in energy, and an onslaught of planning and thoughts about the future. It may seem like a time when meditation would be incredibly difficult because of all that is going on in the mind, but many students find that mindfulness practices are hugely helpful for slowing down their thoughts and helping their nervous system reach a calmer state. As teachers, we also have the opportunity to use meditations to address students' worry and anxiety, which may be part of their experience of being pregnant or in approaching labor and childbirth.

I encourage you to craft and create meditations that work for you as a teacher and that resonate with how you teach and offer prenatal yoga to your students. What you'll find in the offerings below is that I avoid meditations on pregnancy being a "wonderful" or "beautiful" thing. For many folks, pregnancy is a trying and challenging time, whether they are experiencing discomfort and pain, facing an unplanned pregnancy, or have found that pregnancy has triggered past traumas. Part of the goal of mindfulness is to help the nervous system to unwind, so choosing our words with thought and intention to create inclusivity for all experiences can help ensure all students feel welcome and at ease during the meditation.

In order to avoid inadvertently triggering students, when designing your meditations, consider the following:

- For some folks, the journey to becoming pregnant was very difficult and may have involved various interventions like IUI or IVF. Students may feel cautious, worried, or even scared about finally being pregnant.
- Many folks experience pregnancy loss, and for many people, miscarriages continue to be at the forefront of their minds. They too may feel some trepidation about pregnancy and worry about baby.
- Emotions and memories associated with sexual trauma and abuse can be triggered by pregnancy and the approaching birth of baby. Some people will not feel safe in their bodies, particularly considering how much attention their bodies may be attracting now.

- Childhood family dynamics, trauma and abuse, or the loss of a parent can impact students and how they perceive becoming a parent or what being a parent means.
- Pregnancy doesn't always feel good. People aren't always excited, and many people find their bodies to be incredibly uncomfortable and strange.
- Recall the inclusive language around gender from Chapter 4 when creating meditations for students.

A Meditation for Worry, Fear, Anxiety, or Stress During Pregnancy

This practice can be done seated or lying down, whatever students find most comfortable. Ensure that if students are lying down, there are props like pillows, blankets, or bolsters to support them. Once they find a comfortable position to sit or lie in, ask them to let the eyes close if that feels comfortable and follow the steps of the practice.

Guide students through the following practice:

(Allow them to stay with this first imagery for 2-4 minutes.)
Notice your breath. Pay attention to the inhalation and exhalation, and feel your breath entering and leaving your body. Now imagine waves at the ocean rolling into shore and out to sea. As you inhale, imagine the breath is like the wave rolling into shore, and as you exhale, imagine your breath to be that wave rolling out to sea. Inhale, wave rolls in. Exhale wave rolls out.

(Again, for 2-4 minutes.)
Now bring the focus to the exhalation, the wave rolling out. Start to gather up in your mind anything you'd like to let go of: stress, worry, fear, body tension, pain, discomfort. See that with each exhalation anything that is there is released. See those things traveling out to sea on the wave of breath.

(Again, 2-4 minutes for the following imagery.)
Move the attention next to the inhalation, the wave rolling in. With the next several breaths start to imagine anything that you need: calmness, energy, relaxation. See those things traveling into the body just like waves traveling into shore from the sea.

(To end, have them stay for 10-20 breath cycles or, if transitioning to Savasana, have them focus on the breath until they are ready to stop the practice and drop into relaxation.)
Once you feel complete, return to your inhalation and exhalation, let go of the imagery and simply watch your breath traveling in and out of your body. Before you open your eyes, notice how you feel.

A Meditation to Prepare for Birth

This practice can be done seated or lying down, whatever students find most comfortable. Ensure that if students are lying down, there are props like pillows, blankets, or bolsters to support them. Once they find a comfortable position to sit or lay in, ask them to let the eyes close if that feels comfortable and follow the steps of the practice.

Guide students through the following practice:

Notice your breath as it moves in and out of your body. As you become aware of your breath and its movement, notice how it happens without you having to think about it or do anything to make it happen. The body is simply breathing in and out, and your mind doesn't have to tell it what to do.

(Allow them some time to notice the breath.)

Now see if you can notice anything deeper. Are you aware of the beat of your heart? Of the movement of your blood in your veins? See if you can notice all the subtle things happening in your body.

(Allow them some time to notice anything else happening in their body.)

There is a deep inherent wisdom to the body. There are natural processes taking place, and the body knows how to make them happen. Whether it's the movement of our breath in and out or the birth of our baby, our body knows what to do. It's only our mind that thinks it can tell the body to do something different. Our goal in birth is to trust the body's wisdom. Whatever our birth looks like, there is always room to trust the wisdom of the body. Whether it's simply trusting that our next inhale will follow the last exhale or that if we persevere, we'll meet our baby.

(Allow them 10-20 breaths to sit with this.)

For now, come back to watching your inhale and exhale. Notice as your breath moves in and out of your body, and trust that you will keep breathing and that your body knows what to do.

A Meditation for the Cycles of Pregnancy

This practice can be done seated or lying down, whatever students find most comfortable. Ensure that if students are lying down, there are props like pillows, blankets, or bolsters to support them. Once they find a comfortable position to sit or lie in, ask them to let the eyes close if that feels comfortable and follow the steps of the practice.

Guide them through the following practice:

Start to notice your breath as it moves in and out of your body. Become aware of your inhale and how it fills your body up with breath, how parts of you feel fuller, more expanded. And then also notice your exhale and, as the breath moves out, notice parts of your body that empty of air. Take a few more rounds of breath and, as you do, notice how the breath moves from inhale to exhale and the way the body feels as the breath moves.

The breath can be this powerful reminder of change that is happening all around us. The inhale and exhale can mirror other cycles in the natural world, like the rising and setting of the sun or the changing of the seasons. We might also think about how the breath is a reminder of cycles of our lives.

Pregnancy is its own unique cycle that happens and remembering it as that—a cycle—can be very powerful for you. It can remind us that, just like the breath, things are always moving and changing. We might notice that as our belly grows, and we watch our pregnancy progress. It's a reminder that things in nature do not stagnate. So, when we're feeling overwhelmed with our pregnancy or uncomfortable in our bodies, the reminder that capacity for change is always there can be helpful. What is sore today might not be sore tomorrow, and, in the grand scheme of things, 9 months is a really short period of time.

Likewise, it's a reminder to stay present. Just like we move in and out of breath and things change, your pregnancy will eventually lead to a whole new cycle of becoming a new parent and then watching the cycles of life that your baby begins to go through. Our breath can remind us to stay present as we witness the unfolding changes before us.

For now, simply return to watching your inhale and exhale. And know that as you do, if things feel hard right now, that will change. And know that if things feel good now, stay present. Keep breathing.

A Meditation for Protection

This practice can be done seated or lying down, whatever students find most comfortable. Ensure that if students are lying down, there are props like pillows, blankets or bolsters to support them. Once they find a comfortable position to sit or lie in, ask them to let the eyes close if that feels comfortable and follow the steps of the practice.

Guide them through the following practice:

Start to notice your inhale and exhale. Become more aware of your breath and notice how your body might start to get heavier as your breath deepens. Now start to visualize yourself surrounded by an orb of golden light. Spend some time envisioning this orb of light as it travels around your entire body, and as you breathe, visualize the orb of light shining brighter and brighter. Visualize this golden field of light kind of like a force field. Any negativity, stress, fear, or anxiety that is directed at you from the outside world bounces of this field and doesn't penetrate it. However, any love, joy, excitement, compassion that is directed at you does travel through. Visualize this golden orb of light protecting you, and inside it you are safe and warm and at peace.

Continue to envision this golden orb wrapped around your body, but now see a second orb of light, this time wrapped around baby. Envision baby floating inside you, not only protected by your body, but also protected by a golden orb of light. Just like the orb of light surrounding you, this orb is a similar force field that will allow all love, joy, excitement, and wonder you have to share with baby to travel through, but any worry, anxiety, fear, or stress you experience will remain outside of baby's sphere. Visualize baby protected and safe.

Now expand your awareness out, see both of you at the same time wrapped in shimmering golden light. Inhale and exhale and visualize that light shining brightly. Know that any time you are feeling worried or stressed or the outside world is pushing worry on you, that you can reimagine these golden orbs of light providing an extra layer of protection for you and baby.

CHAPTER 10

Yoga for Support in Labor and Childbirth

While the majority of students come to yoga during their pregnancy to help navigate the changes in their bodies and the discomfort that comes with them, many students also will be interested in the ways in which yoga can help them prepare for labor and childbirth. I always tell my students there is no magical yoga pose that will make things better when they're in the thick of it during labor. But here's how yoga can be incredibly supportive during their labor:

- Yoga teaches us to connect ourselves to our breath. Through yoga, we can notice how we breathe, when we breathe, and how our breath can help us navigate things that are challenging. Of all the things we talk about in class, the breath is the number one thing students come back again and again and tell me helped them in labor.
- Prenatal yoga focuses on strengthening the body in preparation for labor. A large portion of the poses we offer in prenatal yoga help to strengthen the legs, hips, and glutes. Labor is often long and daunting work, and contrary to movies that portray childbirth, it rarely happens lying on the back 100% of the time. Laboring folks will find themselves walking, squatting, standing, and supporting themselves on hands and knees. The muscles they build in their yoga practice can help support them as they change positions to labor and birth their babies.
- Prenatal yoga teaches connection to the wisdom and strength of one's own body. A great deal of the process of labor is getting yourself out of your own way and trusting your body knows what to do. This comes in the form of intuitive movement, labor rituals, and breath but also in trusting the process even when it feels overwhelming and hard. Yoga offers the opportunity to connect to our bodies and listen to how they want to move, and also to become aware of how inherently strong the body is. The confidence students build in prenatal yoga can directly translate to their labor and birth experience.

- Prenatal yoga focuses on opening the hips and pelvis. While we concentrate on poses that provide stability and support for hips and pelvis that can feel a little more open due to relaxin, prenatal yoga classes also focus on creating space the hips and pelvic region. As students get closer to childbirth, this space can help baby find better positioning, which can ease the transition of baby during labor and birth.

And let me mention here, too, that Cesarean birth is just as hard and just as big of a deal as vaginal birth. The tools we use to connect students to their breath and to understand the strength of their bodies also will be invaluable to students with planned and unplanned Cesarean births.

Now, let's look at some specific tools we can offer students as they get closer to childbirth and enter labor.

Yoga Support for Breech Presentation (and Transverse)

Babies move around a lot in utero. From very early on, the fetus is extremely active, but it's only when baby grows to a certain size—generally between 14 and 18 weeks—that pregnant folks will start feeling baby's movement. Movements initially feel small and, as baby grows, will feel much more intense, though it's not the movements that have changed, but the comparatively tighter space in the abdominal cavity as baby grows. All this movement is normal and part of baby exploring their environment. Something else that's normal? Some babies switch their position from head up to head down throughout pregnancy.

Often times, babies will settle in to head-down position relatively early. The head is much heavier than the rest of the body, and babies are naturally pulled this direction by gravity, due to the head's weight. If baby prefers to be head up or transverse (sideways), it won't really become a concern until 32-34 weeks. Until that point, baby has a fair amount of room to move around and reposition themselves before childbirth. Keep this in mind, as some students will get a diagnosis of breech presentation earlier in their pregnancy, which isn't necessarily indicative of baby staying in that position for the remainder of pregnancy or birth.

For those who do have a baby in breech or transverse position around the 32-34-week mark, there are many things they can do to encourage baby to flip position. With that in mind, sooner is better for beginning non-invasive interventions like yoga to encourage baby to move. So, invite students to let you know in that 32-34-week time period rather than waiting till 39 weeks to ask how yoga might help to flip a breech or transverse baby.

What is Breech Presentation?

Breech presentation is when baby's feet are facing down instead of baby's head. Head down is ideal for birth, as birthing with baby's feet first is more challenging and requires a provider who is practiced and confident in delivering breech babies. And while they are few and far between, at least here in the United States, there are some out there. If vaginal birth is something a student is interested in exploring, they can try to seek out a provider in their area who delivers breech babies.

A Note on Transverse Babies

Transverse describes babies who are, in essence, lying sideways in the womb. This can be quite uncomfortable for the pregnant person as baby starts to get bigger. While transverse babies will often flip to head down, they also can flip to breech, so use these options for breech presentation to help move a baby in transverse position as well.

Tips for Breech Presentation

If a student is open to them, the following non-invasive techniques have been shown to help babies flip. Advise them to seek out a provider who specializes in working with pregnant folks and has had experience working with babies in breech presentation:

- Acupuncture
- Chiropractic (find someone who does the Webster technique)
- Spinning Babies ®
- Encourage students to get into a pool to swim. Being in the water makes the body more buoyant and requires the body to do less work holding baby and the growing uterus. As a result, hip muscles and pelvis can relax making a little more room for baby to navigate a different position.
- Put cold packs at the top of the belly near the ribs to encourage baby to move away from the cold.
- Play music or have a partner talk at the bottom of the belly by the pubic bone to encourage baby to move toward the sound.

Yoga for Breech Presentation

The goal with yoga poses is to help baby get some space to move around and find more optimal positioning. *Note that none of these poses will flip a baby that is already in head-down position.*

- Downward Dog
- Wide-Legged Forward Fold with hands walked away from pelvis: Much like Downward Dog, but the width of the feet can make this pose attainable for longer periods of time.
- Shoulder Stand at the wall: This can be coupled with Legs Up the Wall so that students can maintain a lift and more space in the pelvis for a longer period of time. This is an intense pose. Students might consider Shoulder Stand for as long as it feels comfortable, then, when it's time to rest, use a bolster or folded blanket to come to

Legs Up the Wall and stay there while they rest. If it feels available later, they could always come back up to Shoulder Stand.

To give baby time to move, encourage students try to stay in positions for an extended period of time. The poses above can be hard to hold for long periods, but the following poses may be more comfortable. Instruct students to come out of the pose and sit up if they start to feel short of breath or like there is too much blood flowing to their head. Otherwise they can stay in each of these poses 5-15 minutes:

- Bridge Pose with the support of a block under sacrum: Get the block as high as possible without losing connection between the feet and the floor. The higher the pelvis goes, the more tip there is to allow baby the opportunity to move out of the pelvic outlet and have more space higher in the abdomen to move around.
- Legs Up the Wall with as much lift under pelvis as possible: The same thing applies here—the higher the pelvis, the better. You may have to slide in a second bolster for students to help lift their hips.
- Meditation/visualization of baby moving into position: It sounds simple, but while students are in these longer poses, have them take time to visualize baby in their belly and visualize them flipping around.
- Avoid deep squatting: We want to minimize anything that encourages baby to drop down into the pelvic bowl any further or to initiate labor.

Yoga Support to Initiate Labor

As students near their due date (and often pass it), the waiting can be the hardest part of the last weeks and days. It's particularly hard, given how much our culture emphasizes schedules—so when things don't happen "on time," we may feel like we're doing something wrong.

The thing is, babies come when they're ready and not a moment sooner. The waiting for baby to arrive will be one of the first of many lessons for new parents about patience and how babies and kids do things on their own schedule, which often has very little to do with what a parent wants.

A teacher friend of mine used to say it was best to think about their due date more like a due month. Baby can come up to three weeks before the due date and up to nearly two weeks after. And ALL of this is within the realm of normal. Given that roughly 5% of babies arrive on their actual due date, it sometimes feels silly that we put so much emphasis on that particular day. Another thing for students to keep in mind is that, generally, first babies will come after their due dates, with subsequent babies often arriving a little earlier than the previous ones.

With that said, sometimes baby's delay in finding the optimal position is what keeps labor from beginning. There are a few yoga poses you can use to help students make more space in the pelvis and encourage baby to shift. Note that none of these poses are going to bring on labor in someone where labor is not ready to start.

Open the Pelvic Outlet

Poses that help open the pelvic outlet are key to making more space for baby to move around and drop into position. A great deal of yoga poses help create space in the pelvic outlet, so know that simply doing their yoga practice will help both student and baby.

- Gate Pose with the hands on the floor and hip circles: This particular pose is hugely helpful. Start in Gate Pose and lower the hands down to the floor directly underneath the shoulders. Ensure the knee is bent over the ankle and the toes are turned out an angle. Then draw circles with the hips (as much as low back and hips allow) in both directions for at least 5 breaths each way.
    - This pose can make pubic symphysis pain worse so avoid this pose if it triggers pain in the pubic region.
    - You can also share with students that this pose can also be a helpful pose for early labor as baby is still shifting position and poses like this can sometimes help address back labor and stalled labor.

Deep Squats

Squats help to create opening in the pelvis and encourage movement of the baby down and into position. These squats are best done from standing, and the depth can depend on what the knees allow. Students might consider squatting with the back at the wall to support balance, which also can give them the opportunity to slide down to a seat to rest after the work of squatting.

- Squat with feet parallel to make more space for baby's head. Feet parallel actually opens the pelvic outlet further than when feet are turned out.
    - This can be particularly helpful in labor if the birthing person is squatting during birth using a squat bar or birthing stool for support. Squat bars can help with getting into a deeper squat, supporting the knees, and be helpful for balance as standing with feet parallel can be a little trickier for some bodies.

Pelvic Rocks at the Wall

Doing pelvic rocks at the wall is a super simple pose that, again, is a movement that can help reposition baby. This is a lot like pelvic rocks done lying on the back, but generally lying on the back won't feel comfortable around 40 weeks.

- Have students come to stand with the back to the wall then walk feet hip-width apart and away from the wall about two feet. Allow the knees to bend a little, then bring focus to the low back. As they inhale, cue to tip the tailbone toward the wall and allow their low back curve to increase. As they exhale, cue to lift the pubic bone toward the ceiling and allow the low back to flatten toward the wall. Continue to rock the pelvis with the breath.

Yoga and Labor

For the most part, in a great deal of Western society, birthing people have never witnessed a child being born before they actually go through our own labor and birth. This can leave the image of childbirth up to the media and the imagination's own worst renderings. As a result, one of the things often feared most about birth is the unknown; a close second is generally pain.

One of the things that can be helpful in exploring pain is to reframe it in the form of sensation. For most of us, pain is a very loaded word. But sensation can be intense or mild, just like pain, and can be a less intimidating way of reframing pain so that we can get a better grasp on the feelings of labor. The second is to understand that a great deal of sensation (or what we might think of as pain) in labor actually has a purpose. It's happening for a reason, and sometimes knowing that reason can help us navigate the intensity of sensation more confidently.

Here are some things that increase sensations we feel in our body during labor:

- During contractions, there is a reduced oxygen supply to the uterine muscles. This reduction in oxygen supply produces waste products such as lactic acid, which can cause muscular discomfort similar to that experienced by runners or other athletes after an intense workout. This often disappears after a contraction ends.
- As the cervix dilates, it stretches out. Without dilation, it is impossible for labor to progress, but the stretching can be uncomfortable.
- As baby descends, there can be pressure on the nerves on or near the cervix and coccyx. Some pregnant folks may have already felt shooting nerve pains during their pregnancy, but they may increase during labor as baby gets closer to the vaginal opening. This sensation, however uncomfortable, signifies that they are getting closer to baby's birth.

- The stretching of the ligaments of the uterus and pelvic joints is a sensation they may have already experienced during pregnancy, but it may be more intense during childbirth. This sensation of stretching plays an important role in making more room in the pelvis for the descent of baby.
- The pressure that baby puts on the urethra, bladder, and rectum can be intense. This sensation signifies that baby is descending the birth canal and they're getting closer to the final stages of birth.
- The stretching of pelvic floor and vaginal tissue as baby begins to crown may be some of the most intense sensation of childbirth. But talk about sensation for a reason— this one means they're about to meet their baby.

Yoga Support for Birth

Yoga is amazingly helpful and effective to help address so many of the aches and pains of pregnancy. It also offers students the opportunity to connect with their ever-changing body and emotions. People often look to yoga to help support them during birth as well.

The thing is, there is no specific yoga pose that will be helpful in birth. What yoga can do is help teach students how powerful their bodies are, it can help to strengthen the body in preparation for the physical needs of birth, and it can help students connect to their breath.

CONNECT TO THEIR BREATH

The breath is the one thing that will be there with someone from the start of their labor to the birth of their baby—and also into new parenthood to boot, which definitely calls for some deep breaths from time to time! Breath is the number one thing students have told me that they have taken from their yoga practice into childbirth—no complex yoga poses, no meditations or mantras, just breath.

You can start this connection to breath a number of ways in your classes:
- Link the inhales and exhales to movement in poses. You might offer a flow in and out of Warrior II and, as you do, cue students to connect that flow to their breath.
- Offer the practice of Sama Vritti. Match the inhale to the exhale, allowing them to become the same length. Encourage students to do this slowly over time and to stop if they notice they feel lightheaded or short of breath.
- Practice lengthening the exhale. Any time we can lengthen the exhale against the inhale, we can help calm the nervous system. Start with the Sama Vritti practice and encourage students to gradually let their exhale lengthen in comparison to the inhale. Again, if they notice lightheadedness or shortness of breath, it's important to stop.

CONNECT TO THEIR STRENGTH

Our own strength can surprise us sometimes—nowhere more so than in childbirth. However, it often takes physical exertion, like a yoga practice, to help students understand their own strength and how they can push through something, even when it is physically demanding or difficult.

Here are some ways to help students connect to their strength in class:

- Invite students to explore staying in yoga poses longer than they think they can.
  - In poses like Warrior II or a Squat at the wall, there is a foundational support for the body. For most bodies, these are poses that can be held for longer periods of time. Pick something stable that can be modified to find more support if needed.
  - When they're in one of these poses, have them notice when their body tells them it's time to come out (this might show up as trembling or a sense of exhaustion or tiredness in the muscles) and invite them to see if they can stay a few breaths longer than they think they can. Students often will be surprised at how much longer they can hold.
    - Make sure to give students the option to come out if they are feeling legitimate pain or that the pose is no longer appropriate for their body.

When we encourage students to stay in difficult poses for longer periods of time, this also gives them the opportunity to practice different forms of managing the sensations they're feeling. When students are in a pose causing intense sensation (we might offer the analogy to a contraction), they can manage the sensation by turning their mind to something else. If they keep their minds busy and focused on something else, the brain has less bandwidth to focus on telling them they're in pain. And this exploration will tie directly into their labor and how they are able to manage pain during labor. Here are a few ways we might offer a different focus for the mind in yoga poses or in preparation for that same practice in labor:

- *Visualizations*: Visualizations can be anything, and different things will work for different folks. Feel free to have them explore their own ideas of what might work, or offer them one of the following:
  - Imagine themselves floating in a pool, their body calm and relaxed.
  - Visualize the sensation in their body like an ocean wave. As the sensation intensifies, imagine the wave rising and peaking. Then as the sensation ebbs, visualize the wave going out to sea.
  - Have them visualize their baby, seeing them and holding them for the first time.

- *Breath*: You can always bring folks back to breath as a tool. Have them watch the breath as they're holding a pose for a longer period of time. You might have them do one of the following:
    - Simply notice the breath and how it changes. Observing if the breath gets fast or short and then encouraging it to get longer and smoother.
    - You can also have students count their breaths as they inhale and exhale.
    - Encourage students to take more audible breaths to keep themselves connected to their breath. Audible exhales out the through the mouth can be particularly helpful not only in the yoga pose, but also in labor.

- *Mantra and sound*: In yoga, mantras are usually specific chants in Sanskrit that are meant to invoke different energies, pay homage to different deities, or direct oneself into a meditative state. In birth and prenatal yoga, mantras can be very different and very simple.
    - You can offer to students that during labor their "mantra" could be as simple as chanting "out baby out" or "doooowwwwnnn" during a contraction. It might feel silly to them now, but I have been at births where parents have used these mantras repeatedly during contractions, and they have helped to keep parents focused and keep their minds away from the intensity of sensation in a contraction.
    - Encourage students to explore making sounds when they are in a more challenging pose, which can be another really powerful tool. Often during birth, people make sounds they didn't know they were capable of making. These sounds can help them negotiate the challenge that birth presents and can help them feel more comfortable when they do make strange sounds (particularly in a hospital setting where more people are coming and going, and it might not feel particularly private).
        - A great practice is to take the three different sounds of Ohm: "Ah", "Oh," and "Mmm." Have students chant each of these individual sounds while they're in a pose. You can talk about how these are a tie to a powerful Sanskrit word, but they are also the sounds that they might make in labor—and some of the first sounds that baby will start to make too!

CONNECT TO THE ABILITY TO RELAX

Relaxation and labor seem to be polar opposites, right? The trick with labor is to identify moments of relaxation, even in active labor. Between each contraction, there is always a resting period. We might think about contractions as a wave that rises, peaks, and then ebbs.

Following the ebbing of a contraction is an opportunity to rest. The closer contractions get to one another, the shorter this rest period is. But taking advantage of these rest periods can make a world of difference in labor, particularly during longer labors.

It might sound counterintuitive, but one of the ways that we can teach students to drop into relaxation is to notice tension in their physical bodies when they are doing something challenging. In the yoga practice, we can have them notice parts of the body that start to tense up when they're in a pose for a long period of time. And I'm not talking about the parts of the body that are directly involved in the pose, but the unconscious places they tense when navigating something hard. For many people it might be a tightening of the shoulders, clenching of the jaw, or furrowing of the eyebrows. Have them notice these when holding a pose for a long period of time and, as they watch these parts of the body, invite them to soften. Sometimes this softening comes from simply bringing attention to a particular part of the body, but it might also mean they need to move that part of the body a little bit to encourage it to relax.

The more students can relax parts of the body that aren't involved in a yoga pose, the more the physical body can recover quickly when they come out. Practicing this in their yoga practice will help them set the foundation for their body when they are in labor.

PREPARE THE PHYSICAL BODY FOR BIRTH

As I mentioned, there's no magic yoga pose that you can offer students for labor that will make things easier or less painful, but what you can do is offer yoga poses during pregnancy that will help them better prepare the body for labor. I like to think of it this way: You wouldn't go out and run a marathon with no prior training. Practicing yoga in preparation for labor is the same thing. Yoga poses can help build strength and create opening in areas that will be most affected by labor and childbirth. Here are the places of focus where yoga can help prepare our students' bodies for birth:

Opening the hips and pelvis: In general, creating extra space in the hips and pelvic region can be helpful for childbirth, given the expansion that happens in this area to make way for baby's descent and birth. Using poses to open hips and pelvis can prepare the body to open and stretch once childbirth begins. It can also be hugely helpful in creating space to allow baby to maneuver their positioning if they're not in an ideal spot leading up to or during labor. Here are some yoga poses that can help with that:

- Squats
- Gate Pose
- Warrior II
- Pigeon Pose

- Bound Angle Pose
- Wide-Legged Forward Fold

Strengthening the legs: If we look at mainstream media's vision of birth, birth happens lying down. For most laboring folks, however, that is not the case. Labor happens in all sorts of different positions, including side-lying, hands and knees, squatting, sitting, and standing. Doing work to help strengthen the legs can be immensely helpful during pregnancy, as folks start to carry more weight in their bodies. And as they approach birth, having the stamina and the strength to use their legs in labor can be immensely beneficial. Here are poses that will help build leg strength:

- Chair Pose
- Warrior I and Warrior II
- Tree Pose
- Half Moon
- Squats

Deep squats: Squatting in general is a huge part of labor for many people. Some folks find squatting during labor helpful; some people will even birth baby squatting. On a physiological level, squatting creates more space in the pelvic outlet for baby to travel through. Also, when squatting instead of lying down, the alignment of the pelvis and sacrum make it easier for baby to descend and uses gravity as an aid to help birth baby. The tough thing? Squatting for long periods of time is hard! There are lots of ways to do supported squats in labor and childbirth, but building strength in the body beforehand can make a big difference in finding support and ease in those positions later.

PART II

THE PREGNANT BODY

CHAPTER 11

An Overview of the Pregnant Body

As I mentioned in the introduction, the information shared here will be limited in scope in order to offer you information as to how things that are happening in the pregnant body impact the yoga practice and to help you better understand where some common discomforts arise. As yoga teachers, it's important to understand our place. We do not have the training of midwives, OBs, or even doulas. The information offered here will simply help you—and possibly assist you in helping your students—understand the general changes in the pregnant body.

The Reproductive System

Upon conception, the fertilized egg travels down the fallopian tubes, growing as the cells divide until it reaches the uterus. Once the blastocyst (as it's now called) reaches the uterus, it implants in the wall of the uterus, which creates the basic blueprint for the growing fetus. As the pregnancy progresses, the release of hormones in the body triggers the thickening of the lining of the uterus.

Early in the first trimester the placenta also will form; it will provide the support system between the pregnant person and the fetus. Oxygen, nutrients, and hormones are transferred across the placenta from the pregnant person's body into the fetus, and waste is transferred back out.

As the pregnancy progresses, the uterus will expand to make room for the growing fetus. By the end of the pregnancy, the uterus will stretch from the pubic area to the bottom of the rib cage.

The Circulatory System

Starting around six weeks, the blood volume in the pregnant body begins to increase. The increase in blood volume helps to facilitate the transfer of respiratory gases and nutrients between the pregnant person and the growing fetus. Over the course of pregnancy, blood volume will increase to 30-40% more than pre-pregnancy levels, which also prepares the body for the loss of fluids that occurs during childbirth.

As blood volume increases during pregnancy, blood pressure gradually falls, with the largest decrease usually occurring around 16 to 20 weeks of pregnancy. However, by the middle of the third trimester, blood pressure levels often start returning to pre-pregnancy levels.

Blood flow to various organs also increases during pregnancy, and that, combined with lowered blood pressure, leads to more work for the heart. Cardiac output—the amount of blood pumped per minute—increases during the first two trimesters, with the largest increase around 16 weeks. By about 20 weeks, cardiac output is 50% above pre-pregnancy levels.

The Digestive and Elimination Systems

Hormones released during pregnancy—primarily increased progesterone—reduce smooth muscle contractions, which slows the movement of food through the intestines and allows the pregnant person to absorb more nutrients during digestion to support their body and the growing fetus. The progesterone also can impact the stomach valve, which keeps acid out of the esophagus, and which is why so many pregnant folks will experience heartburn, too.

The Endocrine System: Hormones and Their Role During Pregnancy

Hormones play a huge role during pregnancy, initiating so many of the changes that happen throughout. Let's take a quick look at the major players and what they do:

HCG (HUMAN CHORIONIC GONADOTROPIN)

This hormone is produced by the developing placenta. It's the hormone that "tells" the body that pregnancy has occurred—the one that over-the-counter pregnancy tests are looking for. The levels of HCG in the body double every two days in the first 10 weeks of pregnancy. The goal? To ensure the ovaries produce estrogen and progesterone. The bad news? Some doctors credit HCG as being one of the culprits causing morning sickness.

ESTROGEN

Estrogen already ebbs and flows in the body during the menstrual cycles, but over the course of a pregnancy, it can surge to over 100 times its normal level. Estrogen is partially responsible for the roller coaster of emotions many folks feel during pregnancy, but it also has many other jobs: It helps to increase the growth of reproductive tissues and size of uterine musculature; stimulates the development of the duct system and blood supply to breast tissue; and is responsible for increased vaginal mucous, subcutaneous fat, skin pigmentation, and water retention.

PROGESTERONE

Another hormone that rises and falls during the normal monthly menstrual cycle, progesterone is responsible for regulating the condition of the inner lining of the uterus. It also inhibits smooth muscle contractions, impacting digestion and elimination and relaxes the uterus. The effect on smooth muscle contractions also impacts the walls of the blood vessels, causing lower blood pressure and resulting in potential light-headedness and dizziness.

RELAXIN

Relaxin is the top hormone for yoga teachers to keep in mind as they teach pregnant students. This hormone is responsible for relaxing and softening ligaments, cartilage, and the cervix. This becomes super important during labor and delivery. Ideally, the cervix and the pelvis will expand to allow for the passage of baby—relaxin is key here. However, relaxin works on all ligaments; as a result, students might notice a sense of instability in the joints or discomfort in the lower back, particularly around the SI joint, as the ligaments relax. Some people instead notice they feel tighter. This seems counterintuitive, but it is the body's way of protecting the joints from instability. As the joints become unstable, the muscles may brace to try to counterbalance this laxness. It's important to be aware of the effects of relaxin on the body during pregnancy as it also can make students more prone to overstretching.

OXYTOCIN

Oxytocin is sometimes called the "love hormone" because it is released during orgasm, following the birth of baby, and during breast/chestfeeding to help facilitate bonding and connection. Oxytocin is also the hormone that plays the biggest role in initiating the start of labor, which is often why folks are encouraged to have sex or do nipple stimulation to start labor or keep it going if it has stalled. This lovely little hormone generally leads to a sense of well-being and connection, but it also is integral in causing contractions of the uterus during labor and helps the cervix to dilate and stretch. Once baby is born, the oxytocin released during breast/chestfeeding can cause minor uterine contractions that can help with the involution of the uterus and can help limit the amount of bleeding postpartum.

CHAPTER 12

The First Trimester

For many folks, the first trimester means nausea, vomiting, and extreme exhaustion. But beyond that, I often tell my students that the first trimester is so challenging because we have very little evidence (other than feeling awful) that anything is happening. The first trimester is tricky because there is a whole world changing inside their bodies but most of the world doesn't yet know they're pregnant, so students may second guess or diminish their experience.

The first trimester lasts the first 13 weeks of pregnancy. Unless someone is charting their menstruation like clockwork or has meticulously planned their pregnancy, some portion of the first trimester may pass by without notice. For others, whether it's due to careful marking of the calendar and waiting for a missed period or to the immediate onset of the first trimester exhaustion and vomiting, they may know almost immediately.

Physiological Changes in the First Trimester

During this time, there are major changes happening internally. Initially the uterine wall will thicken, and blood supply to the uterus will begin to increase. By about 12 weeks the placenta will be completely formed. Many folks won't notice too many outward changes during this time.

The fetus however, if we could see it, is going through most of the major changes at this time, including developing its primitive nervous system and circulatory system (the heart is beating by the 25th day after conception). In fact, by about the eighth week, the embryo will be structurally complete, and while it might not be something students yet feel, it is extremely active.

What will be evident for most pregnant people during this time are the extreme changes in their internal mental and emotional world: the emotional turmoil that comes at the hands of hormonal changes, combined with understanding the fact that they're pregnant.

Common Discomforts During the First Trimester

The discomforts experienced in the first trimester are mostly a result of the hormonal fluctuations. And while changes might not be visible, the discomforts that result from them are often very intense.

Students may also feel very tentative about their pregnancy during the first trimester. Pregnancy losses can occur for many reasons and happen at a higher rate during the first trimester. As a result, if there is any concern about the viability of the pregnancy or past miscarriages students should err on the side of doing less and do what feels safe for them.

Nausea

Nausea can be one of the greatest challenges many people face in early pregnancy, and for those with extreme nausea and vomiting called Hyperemesis Gravidarum, it can be absolutely debilitating. It is often the reason that students won't attend yoga classes during their first trimester.

The interesting thing about morning sickness is there isn't one identifiable cause. It may be partially due to an increased sense of smell due to rise of estrogen in the body and this sensitivity to smells can trigger nausea. Morning sickness is also linked to increasing levels of HCG. And for others, low blood sugar may also trigger nausea. Regardless of what cause, there are some things that can help keep the nausea at bay.

Tips for Nausea
- Always encourage students to eat lots of small meals and have snacks at hand. They might even consider having food with them by their yoga mat.
- Encourage them to stay hydrated. Have them keep their water by their yoga mat and sip as needed.
- Be aware of scents in your yoga studio space. Avoid using incense or aromatherapy oils, as this can trigger nausea for many people.

Yoga for Nausea
- Avoid lots of up and down or quick movements in the asana practice.
- Advise students to avoid closing their eyes in poses if that makes their nausea worse.
- Offer them calming, soothing poses such as Legs Up the Wall or Child's Pose with a bolster.

Enlarged and Swollen Breast/Chest Tissue

Due to the increased levels of estrogen and progesterone in the body during pregnancy, many folks will experience enlarged and swollen breast/chest tissue as early as the first trimester. For some, the change is slight, similar to changes they might notice during their menstrual cycle. For others, the change can be drastic and will have them scrambling to navigate this new body they're inhabiting.

Tips for Enlarge and Swollen Breast/Chest Tissue
- If they wear one, encourage students to invest in a bra that fits. Make sure they're aware that breast/chest size might change again once milk comes in so its best not to invest in too many.
- Cabbage leaves and cool compresses can help if breasts/chest are feeling uncomfortably swollen.

Yoga for Enlarged and Swollen Breast/Chest Tissue
- In the first trimester, it's considered OK to lie on the belly, as long as students feel comfortable. If they are on their belly in poses like Cobra, give them options like Sphinx Pose to take pressure off the chest and offer stacked fists, instead of stacked palms, when they are resting their heads on the floor between poses.
- If students aren't comfortable in poses such as Downward Dog, advise them to stay in more neutral positions like Cat/Cow.

Frequent Urination

We might think the urge to pee all the time doesn't start till baby gets really big, but it can start right away for some students. Early in pregnancy, the kidneys will begin working harder to process not only the waste of the pregnant body, but also the waste of the growing fetus. In addition, the uterus puts pressure on the bladder as it increases in size. All of this combines to create a state of constantly needing to pee.

Tips for Frequent Urination
Unfortunately, there are no yoga tricks to help students navigate this side effect. Ensure they continue to drink lots of water during class to stay hydrated, and encourage them to use the restroom during class if they need to.

Fatigue

Fatigue comes in many forms throughout pregnancy. For many folks, it hits in the first trimester and rears its head again in the third. Increased levels of progesterone in the body are responsible for first-trimester fatigue. And while students might not actually be able to see much just yet, there is a lot going on internally as the body works hard to support the developing fetus.

Tips for Fatigue

It seems counter-intuitive, but regular exercise can make a big difference in bolstering a student's energy. Encourage them to come to class even if they're feeling tired, or help them find classes that are lower intensity or restorative so they can move at a pace that matches their energy levels.

Yoga for Fatigue
- Restorative Yoga practices are a great way to get moving while still honoring the need for rest. Offer students restorative poses in class as an alternative to sequences that aren't as friendly to the pregnant body.
- One of my favorite yoga poses for fatigue is Legs Up the Wall. This pose is great when energy is low, and it also can alleviate swelling and provide support to the female reproductive system through increased blood flow to the pelvic region.
- Yoga Nidra practices can be of huge help in supporting the fatigue.

Constipation/Gas

We may think this fun little side effect of pregnancy wouldn't show up until the third trimester when baby is taking up a great deal of space in the abdomen and pressing on the internal organs, but for many folks, it shows up right away in the first trimester. Increased levels of progesterone slow down the soft muscle contractions of the intestines, which slows digestion so more nutrients can be absorbed. When food moves more slowly through the digestive tract, constipation and gas are natural side effects.

Tips for Constipation/Gas
- Encourage students to increase their fluid intake. This is a great practice regardless, but in pregnancy it can be especially helpful in relieving constipation and gas.
- This is another area where regular exercise can help. Encourage students to attend yoga classes or find other forms of exercise that keep them moving.
- You can suggest that students experiencing constipation or gas supplement their diet with more leafy greens and fiber, which can help support elimination and meet some of the increasing nutritional needs of the pregnant body.

Yoga for Constipation/Gas

It is still okay for students in their first trimester of pregnancy to be on their backs for extended periods of time. This series of poses can help stimulate elimination and support the release of gas in the body:

- Pull knees to chest for 5 breaths.
- Keep right knee hugged in and extend left leg for 5 breaths.
- Switch, hugging left knee in and extending right leg for 5 breaths.
- Alternate between the two for 3 rounds.
- Pull both knees to chest when complete.
- Widen knees and take Happy Baby Pose, stacking feet over knees and holding back of thighs, shins, or feet for 15 breaths.

Headaches

Headaches are a less common side effect for many newly pregnant students, but those who do suffer from them may find them incredibly challenging. The surge of estrogen that comes with the onset of pregnancy, combined with increased blood volume in the body, is often responsible for triggering headaches.

Tips for Headaches

- Encourage students to try prenatal massage. Sometimes neck and shoulder tightness can trigger headaches, and massage may help release those muscles and possibly alleviate the pain.
- If headaches are significant and ongoing, suggest that students contact their care provider to inquire about prescriptions or pain medications to help relieve the pain.

Yoga for Headaches

- Unfortunately, there are no miracle yoga poses for headaches brought on by hormonal changes, but encourage students to avoid poses that may trigger them. Any pose where the head is below the heart can trigger headaches, including:
  - Downward Dog
  - Forward folds
  - Legs Up the Wall
- Some headaches may be exacerbated by neck and shoulder tension. Explore neck stretches that might help release tension in that area.

Low Back Pain

This is something that will follow students throughout pregnancy, but many are surprised when it happens so early. In the first trimester, it isn't so much the change of posture as baby grows that causes pain; it's more due to the hormones released in early pregnancy.

Yoga for Low Back Pain
- Cat/Cow is one of my absolute favorite yoga poses for low back pain. It's intuitive and accessible, and it can feel so, so good! When teaching Cat/Cow, focus on the arch of the back into the Cat spine. Students will also find flowing from Cat back into Child's Pose will allow for a stretch for the low back.
- Downward Dog early in early pregnancy can help lengthen muscles in the low back.

Mood Changes

For so many people, pregnancy is a roller coaster of feelings from day one. The mere experience of becoming pregnant, being pregnant, and thinking about life with a new baby can be enough to make one's mood swing from elated to overwhelmed in a moment. On top of processing this huge life change is the giant hormonal cocktail of mood-altering estrogen and progesterone. Folks may find they cry, feel angry, or get frustrated at the drop of a hat.

While the hormonal roller coaster can feel out of one's control, it is possible to manage the side effects that can influence mood like fatigue and metabolic changes. Ever noticed how your fuse is shorter when you're exhausted? Fatigue can definitely affect the mood. And hangry (hungry + angry) has a whole new definition during pregnancy.

Tips for Mood Changes
- Encourage students to continue with their yoga routine, as the combination of movement and stress relief offered can be amazingly beneficial to support mood changes. In fact, any exercise can make a big difference.
- Tell students not to discount what their bodies tell them. Keeping hunger and fatigue at bay does wonders for keeping mood changes in check! Snacks and naps are key throughout pregnancy.

Yoga for Mood Changes
- Breath practices can help calm the nervous system and relieve stress. Try these two breath practices:
    - Balancing the inhale to the exhale
    - Longer exhalations to inhalations

- Encourage students to take longer Savasanas, or build them into your class (10 minutes is definitely not too long).

CHAPTER 13

The Second Trimester

Beginning in the 14th week and going through the 26th week, the second trimester is sometimes called the "honeymoon" period. And for many people it is: Nausea and morning sickness often diminish, energy often returns, and baby hasn't put on significant weight yet to cause some of the back pain, discomfort, and general claustrophobia that the third trimester can bring. That said, it's not always a honeymoon for everyone and sometimes the second trimester's sense of ease doesn't kick in till the 16th or 18th week—or ever.

In general, people in their second trimester of pregnancy will have more energy to do some of the things they love. For most, baby will start showing a little—or a lot—during this time, and folks will feel more comfortable letting you know about their pregnancy. Some of a student's worry about their pregnancy may also abate after they make it through the first trimester as miscarriages are less likely in the second trimester. Which can be of relief to those who have experienced pregnancy loss in their journey to this pregnancy. For all of these reasons, the second trimester is often when you will see students return to your regular yoga classes after first-trimester trials kept them away. This is also when people tend to begin prenatal yoga classes.

Physiological Changes in the Second Trimester

The second trimester is when students' pregnancies will most likely begin to show. The uterus is expanding in the abdominal cavity in response to the enlarging fetus and placenta and increased amniotic fluid; as a result, the belly is starting to expand.

On this note, it's important for teachers to remember that every body is different and every pregnancy is different. Some people show early on in their pregnancies, and others don't show till well into their second trimester. So much can affect this: height, how the uterus rests in the body, the amount of weight gained, the amount of fluid the body takes on, and many other factors.

What's going on with the fetus? The organs and structures that formed in the first trimester begin to enlarge and mature. Their hair, eyelashes, and eyebrows start to appear, and so does lanugo, a fine, downy hair on the fetus's arms, legs, and back. (Most babies lose some or all of this lanugo hair before they are born. Those who still have some when they're born will slowly lose it over time.)

Common Discomforts in the Second Trimester

You'll find that during the second trimester folks often report less in the way of physical discomforts. The second trimester is a time when the nausea and fatigue of the first trimester has often passed, but the musculoskeletal discomforts of the third trimester have not yet arrived. That being said, there may still be certain discomforts that arise and those listed below may also show up in the third trimester as well.

Gastrointestinal Slowing, Heartburn, and Indigestion

Digestive issues are a result of a combination of things, namely the expanding of the uterus and lower HCl and Pepsin levels, which contribute to the indigestion and heartburn common in the second and third trimesters of pregnancy.

Hormones play a huge role in gastrointestinal issues during pregnancy. As pregnancy progresses, the increased levels of progesterone slow the muscular contractions of the intestines so more nutrients can be pulled from the food before elimination. And the hormone relaxin relaxes the sphincter between the stomach and the esophagus, allowing acid that is supposed to stay in the stomach to make its way up into the throat. This causes heartburn or acid reflux, particularly when folks lie down.

Tips for Digestion
- Encourage students to eat small meals more often throughout the day. The less the body has to digest at once, the better. These same principles are also part of Ayurveda, yoga's sister science. Ayurveda additionally suggests avoiding eating spicy foods that increase "pitta" or heat, which manifests in this case as heartburn.
- Invite them to talk to their care provider about a digestive support like papaya enzymes. If folks are extremely uncomfortable or their heartburn is keeping them from eating, there are higher strength medications a care provider may prescribe.
- If symptoms worsen at night, advise them to position their head a little higher than their belly. This can mean propping the pregnant person up with pillows or, for some folks in a bad place, putting lifts underneath the head of the bed, tipping the whole

bed so the pregnant person can sleep upright in order to keep everything in the stomach and out of the throat.

Yoga for Digestion

- Avoid poses like Downward Dog where head is below the stomach, which can trigger heartburn. Instead give students options to stay in Cat/Cow or do right angle at the wall.
- Other poses like Child's Pose also trigger digestive issues. Sometimes offering stacked fists or putting a bolster under a student's head and chest to keep their head in line with or above their stomach can help. If this still triggers symptoms, invite them to stay with Cat/Cow.

Lightheadedness/Dizziness

By the end of the second trimester, blood volume will have increased over normal levels by 30-40%! The increase helps better support baby's needs as they grow, but it's also in preparation for blood loss during childbirth. With this increase in blood volume, pregnant folks generally will see a decrease in blood pressure and a 10-15 % increase in heart rate. The impact on the circulatory system is huge and can contribute to lightheadedness and dizziness in pregnant folks at this time.

Another factor? As baby grows, they take up more and more space in the abdominal cavity, pushing internal organs up and into the diaphragm, which diminishes lung capacity and sometimes even affects the ability to take deep breaths.

Yoga for Lightheadedness/Dizziness

There aren't any special poses to help students here, but there are a few things to keep in mind:

- If students' dizziness doesn't pass, get them to the floor to rest in Child's Pose, savasana with the support of props, or legs up the wall.
- Cue coming to standing slowly. Consider pausing in a Squat with the head higher than the heart before coming all the way up.
  - For some students, coming up on the exhale can help them avoid lightheadedness as they come to stand.
- Be aware of the breath cues as a teacher. Generally, pregnant students will not be able to breathe as deeply or slowly as they did before they were pregnant. Shorten your cues when teaching to prenatal students.
- If you have a pregnant student in a regular vinyasa class with a lot of ups and downs, such as a series of Sun Salutations, give them alternative options. Sometimes a lot of

fast movement between standing poses and poses with the head down, like downward dog or forward fold, will trigger lightheadedness and dizziness.

Congestion

For some pregnant people, the increase in progesterone combined with increased blood flow to mucus membranes can leave them feeling stuffed up and congested. The technical term for this is pregnancy rhinitis, which may feel like intermittent allergies throughout pregnancy.

Tips for Congestion
Since some traditional Western medication for congestion isn't considered safe for pregnant bodies or the growing fetus, encourage students to try using a Neti Pot. This is just one practice from Ayurveda, the sister science of yoga, which offers many healing remedies that can be helpful during pregnancy.

Muscle Cramps

Muscles cramps can be the worst, particularly those debilitating middle-of-the-night calf cramps that can simultaneously immobilize people and send them jumping out of bed, trying anything possible to stop the intensity of sensation. Why does this happen? Many things come into play, including the increased weight of pregnancy putting pressure on the legs, decreased blood flow to the legs, and, in some cases, nutritional deficiencies.

Tips for Muscle Cramps
Encourage students to check with their care provider about adding a calcium-magnesium supplement to their diet. Magnesium can help with calf cramps, and a calcium-magnesium combination helps the body more efficiently absorb the magnesium. It's best to take the supplement before bed, as it's also a mild muscle relaxant and can help folks overcome insomnia—an issue some students may experience more in the second and third trimesters.

Yoga for Muscle Cramps
At the beginning of moving into Opposite Limb Extension, have students start in Table Top Pose and extend one leg with the toes tucked on the floor. Push weight into the heel to help lengthen the calf muscle.
- Avoid the cue of pointing the toes in poses, as this can trigger calf cramps.

Placenta Previa

This is not so much a common side-effect as something students may have diagnosed and will share around the second trimester of pregnancy. Placenta previa is when the placenta lies low in the uterus, covering all or a portion of the cervical opening. Placenta peavia puts the pregnant person at a higher risk as they need to avoid pre term labor and if placenta previa is still present close to the due date they will have a scheduled Cesarean birth. Placenta previa creates a risk for hemorrhaging for the pregnant person and risk to the baby during birth.

While this diagnosis is intense, know that for some students, particularly with partial coverage, there is a chance over time that as the uterus expands the placenta will move away from the cervix and then no longer be an issue. And folks who have had a diagnosis will generally still receive clearance from their care provider to practice yoga.

Yoga for Placenta Previa
Students should avoid all deep squats. During any kind of squatting movements in class, have students keep squats extremely shallow.

Gestational Diabetes

Again, not a super common complaint in pregnancy, but something students may metion in circle during their second trimester as gestational diabetes is usually screened for between 24 and 28 weeks. They are not entirely sure what causes it but it may be due to hormones from the placenta that block insulin production. For most students it can be treated with changes to the diet but some may have to use insulin for the remainder of the pregnancy. Gestational diabetes often leads to higher birth weights in babies which may make vaginal birth more difficult.

Yoga for Gestational Diabetes
Yoga is of great benefit to folks dealing with gestational diabetes and there should not be a need to modify practice for this complication.

CHAPTER 14

The Third Trimester

For many people, this is the "are we there yet?" period of pregnancy. The third trimester begins at the 27th week and can last till anywhere from 38 weeks to about 42 weeks.

Physiological Changes in the Third Trimester

Much of the fluid retention and weight gain of pregnancy occurs during the third trimester, and some people start to notice contractions, called Braxton Hicks, particularly toward the end of pregnancy. And just in case this period wasn't feeling overwhelming enough for people anticipating the imminent arrival of a new little one, hormonal fluctuations similar to those they experienced in the first trimester will trigger mood swings and strong emotions, too.

For the fetus, this is the growth period when features such as fingernails, hair, and fat deposits become more refined. Baby begins to experience periods of sleep and wakefulness and respond to bright light. Loud noises may also elicit a reaction, and baby will begin to hear and become familiar with parent(s) voices.

At this time, placental estrogen increases, causing the uterus to become more sensitive to oxytocin. This also causes a release of prostaglandins, which soften the cervix and influence the start of labor.

Common Discomforts in the Third Trimester

This period is one where yoga can be of the most benefit to your pregnant students. Many of the discomforts that happen at this time are the result of the changes to posture, the growth of baby and added weight gain. Musculoskeletal issues will be some of the biggest complaints and fortunately, yoga can be a great support to addressing these. We'll go into the majority of musculoskeletal complaints in the next chapter, but below you'll find some other common complaints during the third trimester.

Difficulty Sleeping

Many students, with the impending due date of their baby on the horizon, feel pressure to squeeze in all the sleep they can, knowing it will be at a premium in the first weeks or months of baby's life. Unfortunately, for several reasons, sleep can be harder and harder to come by for many folks in the third trimester.

First, due to the increased size of baby, it is harder for pregnant people to find comfortable positions to sleep. Baby's weight can put pressure on the pregnant body's joints and pull on ligaments, causing physical discomfort that may wake folks up. Second, pregnant folks may find they're waking up several times during the night to pee, caused by the increased pressure on their bladder as baby grows and the extra waste processed by the fetus and pregnant body. Lastly, their inability to eat large amounts of foods combined with the higher caloric needs of this later stage of pregnancy can cause blood sugar to spike at night, giving pregnant people yet another reason to wake up in the middle of the night.

Tips for Difficulty Sleeping
- Pregnancy pillows can make a huge difference in physical discomfort while sleeping. Encourage students to find one that works for them.
- Suggest that students stay thoroughly hydrated throughout the day but stop drinking water about an hour before bedtime.
- Pregnant folks may find that eating a fatty snack, like a slice of cheese or a handful of almonds, before bed can help keep nighttime hunger at bay. They might also consider keeping a snack by their bed in case they wake hungry in the middle of the night.

Yoga for Difficulty Sleeping
- Hip soreness is one of the top causes of physical discomfort waking students at night. Sometimes hip-strengthening exercises can help. Add Side-Lying Leg Lifts and Clamshells to the practice.
- Long Savasanas can be very relaxing, leading some students—even those experiencing difficulty sleeping at night—to doze off in class. Another reason that they're so important for pregnant folks!
- Yoga Nidra practices can be a huge help for any sleep or exhaustion issues.

Hemorrhoids, Varicose Veins, and Swollen Ankles

These symptoms are listed together because they all have the same root cause during pregnancy: the combination of increased pressure within the abdomen and decreased blood flow to and from the legs. Add the effects of progesterone on relaxing the walls of blood vessels, and varicose veins and hemorrhoids become even more likely. Swelling, especially in the last weeks of pregnancy, is particularly common as the body takes on fluids to help prepare for childbirth.

A quick note on swelling: Most folks experience some form of swelling or another, but if it is accompanied by other symptoms like prolonged headache or changes in vision, this can be a sign of preeclampsia. They should contact their provider immediately.

Tips for Hemorrhoids, Varicose Veins and Swollen Ankles
- Encourage students to seek out prenatal massage therapists, who can be incredibly helpful for alleviating varicose veins and swelling.
- Let students know that swimming can relieve swelling anywhere in the body.
- Encourage students to up their water consumption and reduce their salt intake to lessen swelling.
- Compression socks (and compression tights with support for the labia for vaginal varicose veins) can help many students relieve or prevent varicose veins.

Yoga for Hemorrhoids, Varicose Veins and Swollen Ankles
- Legs Up the Wall is beneficial for students with varicose veins or swollen ankles.
- Advise students suffering from hemorrhoids to avoid deep Squats.

Breathlessness

During pregnancy, folks have a 15-20 % increase in their need for oxygen, as they're supplying oxygen not only to their own bodies but also to the growing fetus. And as baby grows, the internal organs are pushed back and up, leaving less room for the diaphragm to expand on inhale and less room for the lungs to take in breath. This combination can lead to breathlessness, which can be incredibly difficult for students, regardless of their cardiovascular fitness prior to their pregnancy.

Yoga for Breathlessness
As a yoga teacher, be aware of the following:
- If students experience breathlessness, they may also experience lightheadedness. Give them the option to rest if needed.
- Cue coming up to stand slowly.

- Notice the cues you give for breath cycles. Keep them a little shorter than you might for a non-pregnant person.

Carpal Tunnel

Wrist pain and discomfort varies for folks in pregnancy, but it shows up most often toward the end of pregnancy, when increased fluid volume in the body presses on the median nerve in the wrist. This can cause tingling and numbness for some and wrist pain for others.

Tips for Carpal Tunnel
If students notice they tend to wake up in the morning with sore wrists, they may be bending their wrists in strange ways while they sleep. Wearing a wrist brace at night can help them avoid putting pressure on the median nerve while they sleep and may alleviate some discomfort.

Yoga for Carpal Tunnel
- For any hands and knees poses, give students the option to be on their fists or set a bolster or blocks under their forearms.
- Dolphin Pose instead of Downward Dog is another option for wrist pain.

Pelvic Discomfort

As baby gets bigger—which is baby's whole goal in the 3rd trimester—baby will start taking up any and all space left in the abdominal cavity. This often means baby will start to press more on the pelvic floor, uncomfortably stretching muscles and ligaments of the pelvis. In addition, as the body prepares for birth baby will often "drop," descending deeper into the pelvic bowl as baby takes position for birth. Baby might then put more pressure on nerves, causing zinging pain in the vaginal or rectal region. (One of my students called it "vagina lightening," which pretty accurately describes it.)

Tips for Pelvic Discomfort
For some folks, a belly band can alleviate some of the discomfort, as it will help lift the weight of the belly off the pelvic bowl and remove some of the pressure.

Yoga for Pelvic Discomfort
Any pose that gets the hips higher than the torso can alleviate some pressure. Offer students poses like Downward Dog or supported Bridge Pose.

Braxton Hicks Contractions

Braxton Hicks contractions are most common in the third trimester, but for some students can start as early as the second trimester. They are a contraction of the uterus that often feels like a tightening of the muscles of the entire abdomen and can last from 60 seconds to about 2 minutes. These are not contractions that will bring on labor and might be thought of best as practice contractions.

The identifying factors of Braxton Hicks contractions are: they are irregular and non-progressing in their intensity and frequency, generally uncomfortable but not painful and will taper off and stop all together. Braxton Hicks are relatively common but may be triggered by dehydration and more intense physical activity.

Tips for Braxton Hicks
- Encourage the student to rest for several minutes till the contractions pass.
- Invite them to drink water or other fluids to help with their hydration.

Yoga for Braxton Hicks
While there are no yoga poses that will stop Braxton Hicks from happening, encourage Restorative poses to help students rest if they are experiencing Braxton Hicks during class.

CHAPTER 15

Anatomical Changes in Pregnancy and Issues Associated with Them

Due to the impact of hormones, weight gain, and the growth of the fetus and uterus during pregnancy, anatomical changes in the pregnant body are inevitable and often the most major complaints for pregnant students, especially later in the second and third trimesters. Fortunately, yoga has so much to offer folks experiencing these changes and the accompanying discomfort.

Over the course of pregnancy, the thoracic and lumbar spine curvature will change. The center of gravity in pregnant bodies tends to move from the pelvis toward the abdomen. As a result, most pregnant bodies experience an increase in lumbar lordosis—posterior tilt of the sacrum and movement of the head back as the body compensates for increased weight as baby grows. The forward shift of gravity, combined with baby's added weight, has a dramatic impact on balance, especially toward the end of pregnancy. This can show up as a change in gait, the postural sway that many pregnant people will describe as a "waddle."

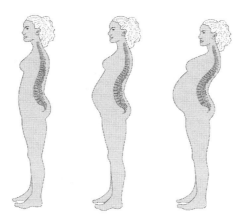

Figure 15.1 The changes to the posture during each trimester.

All these changes to posture can then lead to changes, including the turning out of the feet when walking, the jutting of the ribs forward, the tilting of the pelvis, and the rounding of the upper back. In turn, these lead to discomfort and pain. Luckily, these often can be addressed to some degree with yoga. Let's take a closer look at some of these specific issues.

Low back pain

The start of low back pain attributed to musculoskeletal changes begins around the second trimester (as opposed to the hormonal changes that arise in the first). Change in the body's posture as baby grows bigger and loss of abdominal support in the front as the belly muscles stretch are leading causes for this low back pain. Relaxin also is a factor as it loosens supporting ligaments and tendons around the pelvis which can also force the back muscles to work harder.

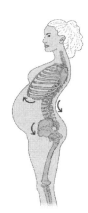

Figure 15.2 Changes to the spine, pelvis and ribs during pregnancy.

Tips for Low Back Pain

- For many pregnant people, belly bands can be helpful in supporting the low back and relieving some low back pain.
- Encourage students to get prenatal massage. For the most part, prenatal massage can help address every single discomfort that comes from anatomical changes. And if they find that regular massage isn't helping enough, working with a PT may be necessary to address underlying misalignment or dysfunction in the body's movement.

Yoga for Low Back Pain

- Cat/Cow is one of my absolute favorite yoga poses for low back pain. It's intuitive and accessible, and it can feel so good for pregnant bodies. When cuing Cat/Cow, focus on the arch of the back into the Cat spine. You also can offer the option of flowing from Cat back into Child's Pose, allowing the seat to come toward the heels.
- In early pregnancy, Downward Dog can help lengthen the low back muscles. Later in pregnancy, it can bring the relief of baby's weight being lifted off the pelvis, which gives the low back a break.
- Pregnant students will start to lose their abdominal support as baby begins to grow in the second trimester, so ensuring they've got other muscles to support the low back is crucial. Strengthening legs, glutes, and hips can help. Offer the following poses:

- o Standing poses like Warriors and Squats can substantially strengthen the legs and glutes.
  - o Side-lying Leg Lifts to help strengthen the hips can relieve a great deal of low back and hip pain.
- Whenever students are in poses like hands and knees or right angle at the wall, remind them to hug baby up and in. This will recruit oblique and transverse abdominal muscles to help hold baby's weight and take some of the load off the low back.

Sacral Pain

The second trimester is when most students start seeing an increase in low back pain, particularly around the SI joint. This is the joint between the sacrum (the heart-shaped bone at the base of the spine) and the ilium bones (the pelvic bones that come around and meet either side of the sacrum in the low back). This is considered a joint because it is held together by connective tissue (tendons and ligaments) and the sacrum can move slightly in relationship to the pelvic bones and may move even more due to the effect of relaxin. During pregnancy, relaxin can cause the joint to loosen and become less stable. Later in the second trimester, postural shifts in the low back, caused by increased weight of baby, put more load on the pelvis, leading to shifts in the hips and, therefore, in the SI joint.

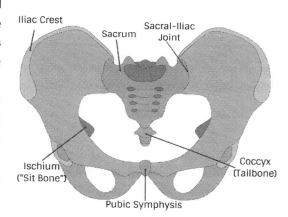

Figure 15. 3 The Bones of the Pelvis

Wondering how to tell the difference between SI joint pain and general low back pain? Students who experience SI joint pain will often feel it on one side but not on the other. It may also show up as sharp one-sided pain that occurs when doing single sided poses that are weight bearing, such as balance poses or even Opposite Limb Extension.

As yoga teachers, making a diagnosis is out of our scope of practice, but it can be helpful to ascertain how and where students are feeling the pain so you can better provide suggestions to help them avoid it in their practice.

Tips for Sacral Pain

- If students are open to chiropractic care, it can be a huge help at this time. Often the hip alignment needs to be addressed, or the sacrum bone needs help finding its alignment. The best chiropractors to see are those who specialize in prenatal care, particularly in the Webster technique. It's great to have a list of referrals of folks in your area who may be able to support your pregnant students.
- Physical therapists can also be of help with this issue. Their focus is more on musculature. A PT may be able to recommend strengthening exercises or stretches for your students that can help with pelvic alignment to take pressure off this joint. Add PTs to your referral list.

Yoga for Sacral Pain

First and foremost, help students avoid anywhere they might be experiencing pain in their practice:

- One-legged poses are generally a big trigger for SI joint pain (but often only on one side):
  - For Opposite Limb Extension on the side where there is pain, have students keep the foot on the floor of the extended leg rather than lifting.
  - Balance poses may hurt on one side, but not the other. Encourage the pose only on the side where there isn't pain.
- Avoid cuing to "square the hips" in Warrior I. This can put extra torque on the SI joint and increase pain in the area.
- Narrow the distance between the feet for Warrior I and Warrior II.

Focus on poses that help create support and containment for the pelvis, which may help mitigate the pain while building muscular support for better alignment. Use a block between the thighs for the following poses:

- Chair Pose can be done, whether simply holding the pose or flowing in and out of it. Consider adding arm variations if students will hold the pose a while.
- Bridge Pose can be done either while holding or flowing in and out. If flowing, consider having students squeeze the block more tightly as they lower down.

Focus on strengthening the glutes to support instability:

- Opposite Limb Extension with leg lifts
  - Use both the options of toes pointing down and turning at the ankle to turn toes to point out toward the long edge of the mat as the extended leg is lifted and lowered.
- Chair Pose, sitting back and squeezing the glutes when coming to stand
- Flowing Squats, keeping feet parallel and squeezing the glutes when coming to stand
- Warrior I, encouraging engagement in the glute of the back leg while holding the pose (often this means focusing on a straight and active back leg)

Sometimes the tightness of the piriformis, one of the deeper glute muscles, affects pelvic alignment. Stretches can help with sacral pain as well.

- Thread the Needle can generally be done early in pregnancy. After about 20 weeks, or once baby makes it difficult to pull the legs in with the hands, try these options:
  - ○ Still on the back, have students place a block underneath the foot of the bottom leg to help draw the legs in.
  - ○ Students can also take the pose at the wall on their backs and use the wall for the foot of the bottom leg.
    - ▪ Note: Have students beyond 20 weeks prop their hips up with a folded blanket when taking either option.
- Pigeon Pose with the support of props can be more intense but will allow students the opportunity to be upright instead of lying down. Ensure they use props to avoid over-stretching and support areas of extreme tightness.

Outer Hip Pain

Outer hip pain becomes a relatively common complaint as students head toward the end of the second trimester and into the third trimester. Outer hip pain can come from a combination of the additional weight associated with pregnancy and baby's growth, increased low back curvature, and loss of abdominal support. These three things cause more work for hips and glutes, as well as a change in how pregnant people walk, which folks often experience late in their third trimester. Toes start to turn outward to help with balance and the extra load of baby. Some lovingly refer to this as the "waddle."

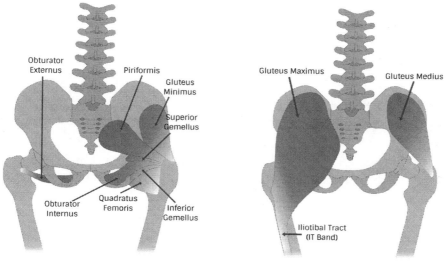

Figure 15.4 Posterior Muscles of the Hips

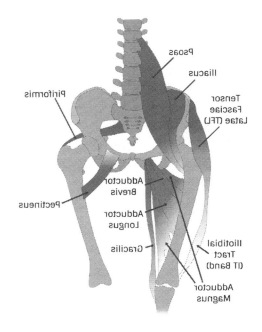

All these things ask much more of the hips, which generally can cause muscle fatigue and strain. Though larger muscles like gluteus medius could provide much more stable support, often small hip muscles like the TFL will compensate and start to take on the bulk of hip support. These smaller muscles tire easily and end up overworked and sore. And with relaxin at play in the body, the tendons and ligaments supporting the hip joint are looser and muscles take over trying to provide support to connective tissues, too, leading to further fatigue and discomfort.

15.5 Anterior Muscles of the Hips

Tips for Outer Hip Pain

- If hip pain is occurring at night, a pregnancy pillow may be able to offer relief.
- Physical therapists often can address issues with outer hip pain. Having referrals for your students can be a great way to provide support.

Yoga for Outer Hip Pain

Generally, when students complain of hip pain, they will ask for stretches to help relieve it. But what often what benefits hip pain like this the most is strengthening the outer hip. Offer the following poses to help address hip pain and provide strengthening:

- Any kind of Side-Lying Leg Lifts or Clamshells
- Leg lifts in Opposite Limb Extension with the toes turned out to the side of the mat rather than pointing down
- Balance poses such as Tree Pose to help them build stabilizing support of the outer hip
- Warrior II

The other area to build strength is the inner thigh. In which case, Side-Lying Inner Leg Lifts will be of benefit. You can also have students use a block between the thighs in the following poses and have students squeeze the block while in the pose or moving in and out of the pose:

- Chair Pose
- Bridge Pose

There are certain yoga poses that may trigger outer hip pain. Encourage students to avoid the following:

- Balance poses on a single side if this position increases pain
- Standing with feet close together. Often standing with feet just a little wider than hip-width apart will make a big difference for those experiencing hip pain.

Pubic Symphysis Dysfunction

For most folks, pubic symphysis dysfunction (sometimes called PSD) shows up in the third trimester, though if students experienced it in a previous pregnancy, chances are good it will show up again (and earlier) in subsequent pregnancies. For most people this shows up as a sharp, shooting pain in the region of the pubic bone.

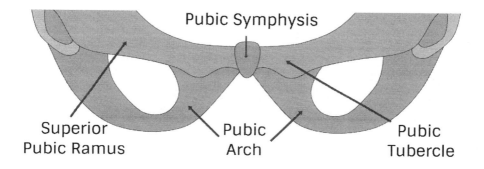

Figure 15.6 The Pubic Joint

It's important to remember the pubic bone is actually a joint. There are two bones that meet at what we think of as the pubic bone and, as with any joint, there is connective tissue that holds it together. And because of relaxin, connective tissue in the body is softening over the course of the pregnancy.

As baby grows, their added weight puts an increasing load on the pelvis, which puts strain on the pubic joint and, for some folks, causes pubic symphysis dysfunction. It will usually show up one of two ways:

1. When doing lunges, after long walks, or following exercise where legs are alternating forward and back
2. When opening the knees away from one another during events like rolling over in bed or getting into or out of the car

Tips for Pubic Symphysis Dysfunction
- Tip number one with any issue related to connective tissue is to avoid doing things that irritate it. The pain is indicative of pressure being point on that joint, generally from more stretching and that is something to avoid if possible.
- Some folks find a belly band to be helpful, as it takes weight off the pelvis and can sometimes lighten the load and the pressure on that joint.
- Be mindful about movements like rolling over in bed. If that is something that irritates pubic symphysis, keep the knees together as much as possible when rolling from one side to the other.

Yoga for Pubic Symphysis Dysfunction
Avoid movements that aggravate it:
- For some folks, deep lunges make things worse, so avoid or shorten the distance between the feet in poses like:
  - Lunge
  - Warrior I
  - Warrior II
- For others, opening knees out to the side worsens the pain, so avoid poses like:
  - Bound Angle
  - Wide Legged Forward Fold (seated or standing)
  - Squatting with toes turned out (suggest Squats with feet closer together and parallel)
- For some balance poses, putting the weight on one side may worsen pain. Avoid those.

Anything that can help create containment and activate the muscles around the pelvis can be helpful:
- Pelvic floor strengthening
- Bride Pose with a block between the thighs
- Chair Pose with a block between the thighs

Sciatic Pain

Often known as sciatica, sciatic pain generally shows up around the third trimester for one of two reasons:
1. **Weight gain:** During pregnancy, increased fluid retention and even the weight of the uterus place pressure on the sciatic nerve.
2. **Increase in low back curvature (lordosis):** This is a result of carrying the weight of baby as they grow. This postural shift can either cause the glutes and low back to

grip, potentially squeezing the sciatic nerve, or pelvic alignment to shift, which also can pinch the nerve.

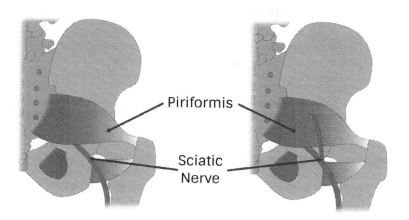

Figure 15. 7 The two variations of sciatic nerve anatomy.

When either of these things happen, the pressure on the sciatic nerve can result in pain that shoots down through the glute and into the leg, for some people, this pain can travel the full length of the leg.

Tips for Sciatic Pain

- Acupuncture, massage, and physical therapy can be helpful in addressing sciatica. It's helpful to have resources to recommend to your students.
- For issues that are more structural in nature, a chiropractor may provide some relief in helping to realign the pelvis.

Yoga for Sciatic Pain

Avoid the following poses as they can make sciatica worse:

- Ardha Hanumanasana
- Pigeon Pose
- The cue of "squaring" the hips in Warrior I

You may need to modify the following poses for students to ensure that the hip alignment doesn't trigger sciatic pain. (If students don't experience pain in these poses, they can continue to do them.) In the following poses, if sciatica is triggered, keep the front foot parallel to the back foot and the leg straight and simply have students take the arm shape of the pose:

- Warrior II
- Triangle Pose
- Side Angle

Round ligament pain

The round ligament is a ligament that holds the uterus in place in the abdominal cavity. As baby grows and the uterus gets increasingly heavy, the ligament must hold more weight. When we combine that additional weight gain of baby in the third trimester with the stretching ligaments under the influence of the hormone relaxin, the round ligament can get overstretched and sore simply holding the uterus in place. Physical activity like walking worsens the pain by forcing the ligament to do even more stabilizing, which is often why this pain shows up after students have walked a long distance.

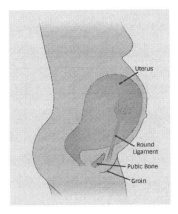

Figure 15.8 The Uterus and Round Ligament

Because most folks aren't generally familiar with the round ligament, they may be uncertain of the cause of the pain until it has been diagnosed by a care provider. Many people find that it feels like a deep ache or sharp pain at the front of their hips or in the groin area that often shows up after longer stretches of physical activity.

Tips for Round Ligament Pain
A belly band can do wonders for round ligament pain, as it takes some of the pressure off the ligaments trying to hold the uterus in place. If folks are experiencing the pain in the mid-second trimester or early third trimester, it's wise to consider a band. If the pain comes on in the last few weeks of pregnancy, getting a band may not be worth it, as the pain will diminish after baby is born.

Yoga Tips for Round Ligament Pain
- Avoid deeper hip flexor stretches like Warrior I. Have them shorten the distance between the feet so they're not lunging into the shape as deeply.
- With round ligament pain, the absolute best thing to do—in yoga or any other activity—is to stop doing anything that triggers the pain.

CHAPTER 16

Changes to the Prenatal Core

Changes to the core are often one of prenatal students' biggest concerns. They're aware they are losing core support and that the belly muscles are stretching, but they are often unsure of what exactly is changing and how it will impact their practice. Most students also have heard about the common risk of abdominal separation (clinically called diastasis recti) during pregnancy but are unaware of what they can do to minimize it or how to heal postpartum.

It is helpful to understand each of the core muscles and their function, so we can better understand how they might be affected by pregnancy and the yoga practice. There are four basic core muscles:

- The rectus abdominis muscle consists of two sets of muscle bellies that run parallel and are held together by connective tissue called the linea alba, which runs vertically from the xyphoid process at the end of the sternum to the pubic bone.

- There are two sets of oblique muscles, which run diagonally down from the ribs (the external) and diagonally up from the pelvis (internal). These are strong support muscles at the side of the waist on the right and left sides of the body.

- The transverse abdominis is the deepest core muscle. It wraps around the trunk, connecting at the spine.

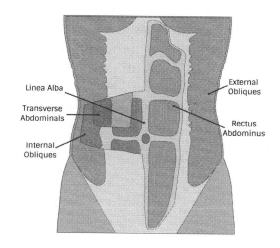

Figure 16.1 The muscles of the abdomen

145

As baby grows, several changes start to affect the core. First, there is the stretching of the muscles, tissue, and skin in the front of the body. Second, there is the added weight carried in the abdominal cavity. These changes are responsible for three significant changes to the body that particularly affect posture:

- The deepening of low back curve, which causes the pelvis to tilt forward and down
- The tilt of the pelvis forward and down, which can cause the low ribs to wing forward, stretch the belly muscles further, and add load on the linea alba, the connective tissue most impacted by diastasis recti—all causing strain on the low back muscles
- Added load on the pelvic floor, which can lead to pelvic floor weakness, impacting overall core function

What is Diastasis Recti?

As mentioned above, the most significant muscle stretching in the core happens along the rectus abdominis and impacts the connective tissue called the linea alba. The linea alba runs along the midline of the rectus abdominis from the bottom tip of the sternum to the pubic bone, connecting the muscle bellies of the abdomen (think of the muscles in six-pack abs). As the uterus expands, the linea alba stretches thin, which can cause the muscle bellies to separate. This creates what is called a diastasis recti, a musculoskeletal injury that occurs when the rectus abdominis tears at the connective tissue, separating it from the linea alba.

Diastasis is worsened when the ribs lift in front, causing stretching in the front and a major shortening of the abdominal cavity in the back. This imbalance can put the contents of the abdominal cavity—the internal organs and uterus with baby growing inside—under greater pressure. This pressure must go somewhere, and because the spine creates a strong, impenetrable boundary in the back, the pressure goes up, down, or forward. Downward pressure weakens the pelvic floor, and upward pressure into the diaphragm can cause reflux. Usually the pressure goes forward because the core muscles provide the weakest barrier, as they have been softening and stretching over the course of pregnancy. The front of the body can only take so much before the muscles can no longer hold it and the connective tissue begins to stretch, causing the separation often experienced postpartum.

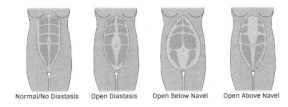

Normal/No Diastasis   Open Diastasis   Open Below Navel   Open Above Navel

Figure 16.2 The Variations of Diastasis Recti

Things Avoid in Prenatal Yoga Classes to Minimize Diastasis Recti

In general, it won't be necessary to avoid anything in the first trimester or even early second trimester. The concern over core work comes as baby starts to grow and the belly starts to expand. Because everyone's anatomy is different, timing will be slightly different. And each pregnancy is different, too. Students may notice their bellies get bigger earlier in subsequent pregnancies than in previous pregnancies. Once significant growth begins:

- Avoid deep twisting, which can put pressure on the linea alba, shearing the rectus abdominis in oppositional movement and straining connective tissues.
    - Offer open twists. For example, in a seated twist, twist away from the bent knee rather than toward it.
    - Base the twists in the upper torso, twisting from the arms and ribcage rather than from the belly.
- Avoid core work like crunches, which shorten the recti muscles and worsens any separation. When the muscles shorten, they bulge out in the middle. Crunches also increases pressure in the pelvic bowl area which can weaken the pelvic floor muscles and contribute to pelvic organ prolapse.
- Avoid most core-based poses like Boat Pose or other traditional abdominal strengthening.
- Cue students to roll to their side and lie down when coming to the floor and roll to their side and press up when coming to a seat.
- Avoid rib thrusting. To find correct rib alignment, instruct students to take the point of the ribcage and move it down and back in alignment with the hip bones. This movement happens at the spine and not with the abdominal muscles.
- Avoid deep backbending and provide support like a bolster under the thighs in backbends such as Upward Facing Dog.
    - Give the cue of "hugging baby in toward spine" to curb rib thrusting.
- Use a block between the thighs for standing poses like Chair Pose and combine with the cue of "hugging baby in" to help students maintain more neutral spine positioning.

Things to Do to Support the Core (and Minimize Diastasis) in Prenatal Yoga

In our prenatal yoga classes, there are several things we teachers can offer that will help students build stronger cores in their pregnancy and also stronger support muscles:

- Use the cue of "hugging baby in" in all poses that ask the core to do some work or that deepen the low back curve.
- Focus on poses that strengthen the glutes and hips.
- Offer pelvic floor strengthening in every class.

Below you will find several poses that can help build core strength during pregnancy:

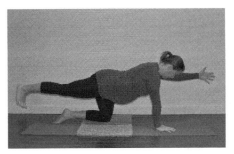

Opposite Limb Extension

Focus on lifting baby up toward the spine.

Keep neutral low back to support the weight of baby in front.

Option to raise and lower arm and leg for added strengthening of the core.

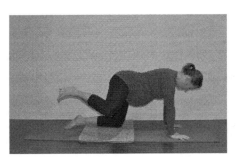

Hydrant Lifts

Focus on lifting baby up toward the spine.

Keep lifting leg bent, with knee bent 90 degrees.

Concentrate not on how high the leg is lifted, but on keeping hips square, which ensures the glutes and hips are engaged.

Maintain balanced weight into the opposite leg and arm.

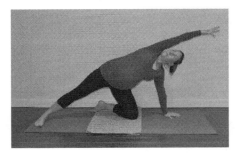

Side Plank Variation

Press outer edge of extended leg's foot into the floor.

Kick foot on same side as bent knee back as far as needed for support of balance.

Reach top arm away from extended leg.

Hug baby in and lift side waist closest to floor toward the ceiling.

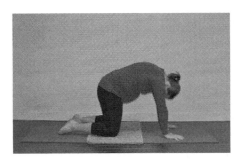

Cat/Cow

Avoid the deep bend of Cow Pose and focus on the arch of Cat Pose (shown here).

When coming to Cat, hug baby toward the spine.

Option to flow back to Child's Pose.

Changes to the Pelvic Floor

It can be helpful to think of the pelvic floor as diamond shape that runs between the four points of the two sit bones, the pubic bone, and tailbone. These muscles create a muscular base to the pelvic bowl, supporting the pelvic organs at the bottom of the pelvis (the bladder, uterus, and bowel as seen in Figure 16.4). We consider pelvic floor muscles to be a part of the broader core because they work in concert with abdominal muscles and low back muscles to help stabilize the spine.

The pelvic floor not only provides support to the organs and the weight of baby when pregnant, but it also gives us conscious control over the bladder and bowel through openings for the urethra and anus. Engaging the muscles allows pregnant folks to delay going to the bathroom, and relaxing the muscles allows the passage of urine and feces. There is a third opening for the vagina which is also lined with muscles like the urethra and anus and can be contracted and lifted as well.

During pregnancy, the weight of the uterus increases, putting more pressure and weight on the pelvic floor muscles. Maintaining strength in the pelvic floor helps to ensure that, as the weight increases, pelvic floor muscles can continue to support the weight of the organs and maintain functionality.

As you can see from the diagram of the muscles of the pelvic floor (Figure 16.3), the openings are part of its muscular sheath. As this whole muscle system bears the extra weight of the growing uterus and baby, the muscles around the openings may start to weaken. As a result, students may notice a decrease in function later in pregnancy when it becomes harder to hold urine in when they need to use the bathroom

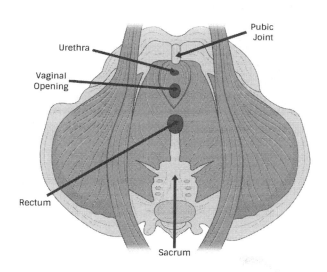

Figure 16.3 Anatomy of the pelvic floor, looking down into the pelvis

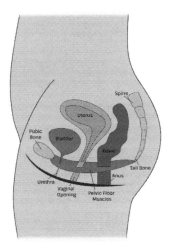

Figure 16.4 Anatomy of the pelvic floor view from the side

Pelvic Floor Lifts

Find a comfortable sitting position. As you begin to work with the pelvic floor, it can be helpful to think of the pelvic floor as diamond shape that runs between the four points of the two sit bones, the pubic bone, and tailbone. It's this hammock of muscles that we want to pull in and up when we exhale. You may find that sitting on a block can be helpful as it can give you awareness of the location of the two boney landmarks of the sit bones.

- Begin by closing the eyes and observing the inhale and exhale for a few breaths.
- On an inhalation, let the pelvic floor muscles soften and relax. It's not a bearing down or a push, just a relaxation.
- On the exhale, pull the pelvic floor muscles in and up. The feeling may be a "squeeze and lift." The pulling in might be thought about as a drawstring bag cinching up around the vaginal opening, and the lift might be found through imagining the pelvic floor muscles as an elevator lifting from the ground floor to the first floor inside the abdomen.
  - o Avoid holding the breath.
  - o Always lift on the exhale to avoid intra-abdominal pressure.
  - o Ensure that glutes and inner thigh muscles are relaxed (though initially you might feel like you are tightening and relaxing your butt muscles).
  - o The sensation should feel like a deep and subtler action.
- Slowly release these muscles on the inhale.

Acknowledgements

This book has been years in the making and as a result, there are numerous people to thank. First and foremost, I offer deep gratitude to all of the students who have journeyed through their pregnancies and postpartum in my classes. You are my greatest teachers. Witnessing the challenges you faced, hearing your struggles, I have learned and grown as a teacher. Thank you for all you have taught me.

Also, a deep bow to Anne Phyfe Palmer, my first Prenatal Yoga teacher. You helped set me on this path of working with pregnant and postpartum students and continue to be a resource and guide for me. I would also like to thank all the Teacher Training trainees I have had the honor to work with over the past years. They say that the best way to learn about something is to teach it yourself. Through your curiosity, questions and inquiry I have learned more as a teacher and I appreciate the excitement with which you all go out into the world to share the gift of prenatal yoga with your students.

Immense thanks to my fabulous editor Madeleine Franti. Without you, this book wouldn't have been possible. You took what I had and made it a hundred times better. Your ability to wordsmith and your eye to structure has helped make this book something I didn't think possible. Thank you, thank you, thank you for all your hard work. You are amazing.

And speaking of amazing, my thanks would not be complete without huge praise for my wonderful and amazing wife Anjelica. Your unending support, love, and belief that I could do this made this book happen. You are always there as my cheerleader and my rock in the craziness of the storm that is currently a toddler and you make me a better person in all things. Thank you for loving me and for believing in me. I love you.

To Sawyer, you have taught me about the experience of pregnancy firsthand, and you remain one of my greatest teachers. You teach me so much about being present, enjoying the simple things, and not taking anything for granted. I am so lucky to be your mama.

To my family, a huge thank you to my aunt, Carol. Your wisdom and insight in navigating the world of self-publishing combined with your love and support helped guide me through this process. And to my parents who always believed I could do anything.

A huge thank you to the friends who have opened up their birthing space to me to be of support as a doula. Thank you to Erin, Laura and Alice for trusting me at this precious time and for showing me the immense power of the birthing body. I am forever grateful.

Lastly, I would like to honor the lineage of yoga and express sincere gratitude for all the teachers who have come before me.

Bibliography

Books and Journal Articles

Bowen, Katy. *Diastasis Recti: The Whole Body Solution to Abdominal Weakness and Separation.* Propriometrics Press, 2017.

Englund, Pam and Rob Horowitz. *Birthing from Within: An Extraordinary Guide to Childbirth Preparation.* Albuquerque, New Mexico: Partera Press, 1998.

Hall, Michael, et all. *The Heart in Pregnancy.* National Library of Medicine, National Institute of Health. PMC, October 2013.

Iyengar, Geeta. *Yoga: A Gem for Women.* Canada: Timeless Books, 1990.

Palmer, Anne Phyfe, et al. *8 Limbs Pre/Postnatal Yoga Teacher Training Handbook.* Seattle, Washington: 8 Limbs Yoga Centers, 2019.

Oster, Emily. Expecting Better: *Why the Conventional Pregnancy Wisdom Is Wrong--and What You Really Need to Know.* New York, New York: Penguin Books, 2016.

Shapirio Bachman, Margo. *Yoga Mama Yoga Baby: Ayurveda and Yoga for a Healthy Pregnancy and Birth.* Boulder, Colorado: Sound True, 2013.

Simkin, Penny, et al. *Pregnancy, Childbirth and the Newborn: The Complete Guide.* New York, New York: De Capo Press, 2016.

Simkin, Penny and Katie Rohs.*The Birth Partner: A Complete Guide to Childbirth for Dads, Partners, Doulas, and All Other Labor Companions.* Beverly, Massachusetts: Harvard Common Press, 2018.

Sparrowe, Linda and Patricia Walden. *The Women's Book of Yoga & Health: A Lifelong Guide to Wellness.* Canada: Random House, 2002.

Online Resources

American College of Obstetricians and Gynecologists, *Physical Activity and Exercise During Pregnancy and the Postpartum Period* (Washington, DC: American College of Obstetrics and Gynecologists, 2019), https://www.acog.org/Clinical-Guidance-and-Publications/Committee-Opinions/Committee-on-Obstetric-Practice/Physical-Activity-and-Exercise-During-Pregnancy-and-the-Postpartum-Period.

Continence Foundation of Australia, *Pelvic Floor Muscles*. https://www.continence.org.au/pages/how-do-pelvic-floor-muscles-help.html.

Statista, Pregnancy- Statistics & Facts. https://www.statista.com/topics/1850/pregnancy.

Yoga Journal, *Yoga in America Study,* https://www.yogajournal.com/page/yogainamericastudy.

Made in the USA
Monee, IL
12 January 2020

20249096R00085